1st EDITION

Perspectives on Diseases and Disorders

Anxiety Disorders

Paul Hina and Sarah Hina
Book Editors

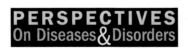

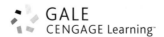

GALE
CENGAGE Learning

Detroit • New York • San Francisco • New Haven, Conn • Waterville, Maine • London

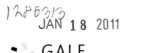
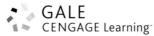

GALE
CENGAGE Learning

Christine Nasso, *Publisher*
Elizabeth Des Chenes, *Managing Editor*

© 2010 Greenhaven Press, a part of Gale, Cengage Learning

Gale and Greenhaven Press are registered trademarks used herein under license.

For more information, contact:
Greenhaven Press
27500 Drake Rd.
Farmington Hills, MI 48331-3535
Or you can visit our Internet site at gale.cengage.com

For product information and technology assistance, contact us at

Gale Customer Support, 1-800-877-4253
For permission to use material from this text or product, submit all requests online at www.cengage.com/permissions

Further permissions questions can be e-mailed to permissionrequest@cengage.com

Articles in Greenhaven Press anthologies are often edited for length to meet page requirements. In addition, original titles of these works are changed to clearly present the main thesis and to explicitly indicate the author's opinion. Every effort is made to ensure that Greenhaven Press accurately reflects the original intent of the authors. Every effort has been made to trace the owners of copyrighted material.

Cover image copyright Paul Matthew Photography, 2010. Used under license from Shutterstock.com.

LIBRARY OF CONGRESS CATALOGING-IN-PUBLICATION DATA

Anxiety disorders / Paul Hina and Sarah Hina, book editors.
  p. cm. -- (Perspectives on diseases and disorders)
Includes bibliographical references and index.
ISBN 978-0-7377-5052-2 (hardcover)
1. Anxiety disorders. I. Hina, Paul. II. Hina, Sarah.
RC531.A593 2010
616.85'22--dc22

2010007130

Printed in the United States of America
1 2 3 4 5 6 7 14 13 12 11 10

CONTENTS

CHAPTER 1   Understanding Anxiety Disorders

Rebecca J. Frey and Teresa G. Odle

A general overview of the various anxiety disorders includes descriptions, symptoms, and available treatment options.

National Institute of Mental Health

Treatment options for anxiety disorders depend on the patients' preference and on their specific diagnosis, but can include medication, psychotherapy, or some combination of both.

Michael L. Nichols

Many people who are affected by anxiety disorders are also affected by depression. The two disorders manifest similar coping strategies in patients and are genetically linked, while also benefiting from similar treatment options.

Mark Rowh

Although the cause of obsessive-compulsive disorder is unclear, the disorder is understood to be brain-based. Treatments include medication and cognitive-behavioral therapy.

FOREWORD

"Medicine, to produce health, has to examine disease."
—Plutarch

Independent research on a health issue is often the first step to complement discussions with a physician. But locating accurate, well-organized, understandable medical information can be a challenge. A simple Internet search on terms such as "cancer" or "diabetes," for example, returns an intimidating number of results. Sifting through the results can be daunting, particularly when some of the information is inconsistent or even contradictory. The Greenhaven Press series Perspectives on Diseases and Disorders offers a solution to the often overwhelming nature of researching diseases and disorders.

From the clinical to the personal, titles in the Perspectives on Diseases and Disorders series provide students and other researchers with authoritative, accessible information in unique anthologies that include basic information about the disease or disorder, controversial aspects of diagnosis and treatment, and first-person accounts of those impacted by the disease. The result is a well-rounded combination of primary and secondary sources that, together, provide the reader with a better understanding of the disease or disorder.

Each volume in Perspectives on Diseases and Disorders explores a particular disease or disorder in detail. Material for each volume is carefully selected from a wide range of sources, including encyclopedias, journals, newspapers, nonfiction books, speeches, government documents, pamphlets, organization newsletters, and position papers. Articles in the first chapter provide an authoritative, up-to-date overview that covers symptoms, causes and effects, treatments, cures, and medical advances. The second chapter presents a substantial number of opposing viewpoints on controversial treatments and other current debates relating to the volume topic. The third chapter offers a variety of personal perspectives on the disease or disorder. Patients, doctors, caregivers, and loved ones represent just some of the voices found in this narrative chapter.

Each Perspectives on Diseases and Disorders volume also includes:

- An **annotated table of contents** that provides a brief summary of each article in the volume.
- An **introduction** specific to the volume topic.
- Full-color **charts and graphs** to illustrate key points, concepts, and theories.
- Full-color **photos** that show aspects of the disease or disorder and enhance textual material.
- **"Fast Facts"** that highlight pertinent additional statistics and surprising points.
- A **glossary** providing users with definitions of important terms.
- A **chronology** of important dates relating to the disease or disorder.
- An annotated list of **organizations to contact** for students and other readers seeking additional information.
- A **bibliography** of additional books and periodicals for further research.
- A detailed **subject index** that allows readers to quickly find the information they need.

Whether a student researching a disorder, a patient recently diagnosed with a disease, or an individual who simply wants to learn more about a particular disease or disorder, a reader who turns to Perspectives on Diseases and Disorders will find a wealth of information in each volume that offers not only basic information, but also vigorous debate from multiple perspectives.

INTRODUCTION

Most people who suffer from a serious illness have a pretty clear-cut path to follow. They pick up their phones, make a doctor's appointment, and seek the professional help they require. And while there might be difficulties and hurdles to face, with regard to treatments and lifestyle changes, these patients usually have the security of knowing that they have done everything possible to protect their future health while also having a valuable support system of family and friends to back them up.

But what if a patient does not know she is sick? Or worse, what if she senses a problem but is too ashamed and terrified to seek the help that is desperately needed? These patients suffer, but they often do so in isolation from the outside world, concealing their illnesses from the very people they love. All too often, these are the patients suffering from anxiety disorders.

Take Diance, a patient suffering from obsessive-compulsive disorder (OCD), one of the many illnesses categorized as an anxiety disorder.

"Forget about dating," Diance said, relating her story to the Anxiety Disorders Association of America (ADAA). "I couldn't touch anybody, I couldn't hug. People would flock around me but I would only let them get so close." And while Diance had been outgoing prior to the development of her OCD symptoms, she eventually stopped socializing with friends and family. She became depressed, in addition to being bombarded by the disruptive, obsessive thoughts that haunted her everyday life. Too ashamed to tell her family of her depression and anxiety disorder, Diance attempted suicide at the age of thirty-five. This was a full ten years after her illness started.

Luckily, Diance's suicide attempt was not successful, and she was diagnosed with OCD by a therapist trained to recognize the symptoms of her disorder. After several years of receiving cognitive-behavioral therapy to break the cycle of repetitive, obsessive thoughts, Diance's social life improved markedly, and she began repairing her broken relationships with family members. Her self-esteem also rebounded. "I'm not perfect. I'm imperfect," Diance told the ADAA. "But I don't hate myself anymore."

It often takes years for patients with anxiety disorders to get help. The lag time between the beginning of OCD symptoms and appropriate treatment may be as long as seventeen years, according to Eric Hollander, professor of psychiatry and director of the Compulsive, Impulsive and Anxiety Disorders Program at Mt. Sinai School of Medicine in New York. What accounts for the delay? "Many people with OCD are ashamed and humiliated by what they consider the bizarre nature of their obsessive thoughts," says Hollander. "Also, they usually recognize that checking or washing or hoarding will not in reality change anything, but they feel powerless to stop. As a result, they are less likely to share their problem with a family member or their doctor."

Another factor contributing to the delay is that OCD may not be the most obvious diagnosis. "Patients often come into their doctor's office complaining of depression or anxiety," says Hollander. "Unless the physician or therapist is thinking about the possibility of OCD, they won't ask the right questions and the diagnosis isn't made."

Diance's strong sense of shame surrounding her OCD is common among patients suffering from anxiety disorders. Like many afflicted with a mental illness, anxiety disorder patients often feel like having a disease "in their head" is a dark secret, the burden of which they are responsible for carrying, and hiding, all by themselves.

Yet by concealing their troubles from others who might help them, they increase their levels of anxiety and delay or even sabotage their chances for recovery.

For patients with social anxiety disorder, this toxic shame lies even closer to the heart of their disease. Most of these patients feel like something fundamental is wrong

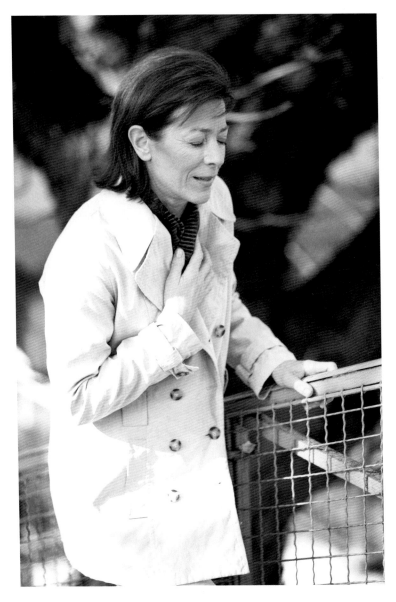

A panic attack comes on suddenly and can be accompanied by hyperventilation, rapid heartbeat, sweating, chest pain, dizziness, and feelings of terror. (Voisin/Phanie/Photo Researchers, Inc.)

with them, something that cannot be fixed. The roots of their poor self-esteem can often be traced to difficult childhood relationships or traumas. They become accustomed to feelings of self-loathing and may even think that they deserve the emotional pain they are experiencing. The only "solution," therefore, is to hide from others and avoid social interactions—where someone might discover their "defectiveness"—at all costs. In a recent national survey commissioned by the ADAA, nearly 90 percent of people said their social anxiety disorder negatively affects their personal relationships, and 75 percent said the disorder affects their ability to carry out normal daily activities. Most of the people surveyed also said they feel as if they are alone.

Often, this shame and isolation spirals into a feedback cycle, in which a patient's self-loathing and anxiety feed on one another to such an irrational extent that full-blown panic might be triggered by perfectly ordinary events. For patients suffering from panic disorder, post-traumatic stress disorder (PTSD), or phobias, this is the central, debilitating pattern of thoughts that isolates them from everyday life. The person's subjective perception becomes too distorted, making him or her unable to understand the difference between a minor problem and a major crisis. Ordinary situations trigger a "fight, flight, or freeze" response. Or, for patients suffering from generalized anxiety disorder, anxious feelings may persist for days with no apparent trigger, while stress continues to build and build. Finally, the individual becomes paralyzed by worry and unable to function normally.

As panic disorder patient Eric Wilinski wrote on his personal blog, "To panic was to be weak, as I saw it then. Panic was something to hide from the world. Since then, as panic, agoraphobia, and depression have caused me to miss important events (weddings, dinner dates, job interviews), lose longtime friends, and fail to build a career I'm very proud of, the shame I feel has only increased."

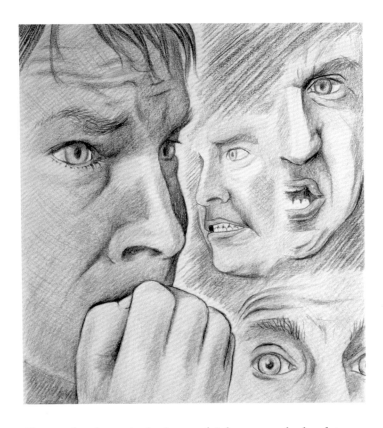

According to the author, people with panic disorders suddenly panic over ordinary events and distort minor problems into major crises. **(Andrew Bezear, Reed Business Publishing/ Photo Researchers, Inc.)**

Shame leads to isolation, which can only lead to more shame and concealment. The cycle eats away at a person's core sense of self and erodes the relationships cultivated over a patient's lifespan.

Fortunately, the dangerous pattern can be broken. Millions of patients with anxiety disorders have taken the courageous step of recognizing that they are ill and not powerless to change their lives for the better. University of Alberta researcher Jessica Van Vliet's study, published in the journal *Psychology and Psychotherapy: Theory, Research, and Practice*, concludes that, while it may seem difficult to escape the cycle of shame, there is great hope for anyone who wants to overcome this harmful emotion.

Van Vliet discovered that one of the key factors in overcoming a deep sense of shame is making connections, be it with family and friends, a religious network, or humanity as a whole. "Connecting to others helps to increase self-acceptance, and with self-acceptance can come a greater acceptance of other people as well," she says. "People start to realize that it's not just them. Other people do things that are as bad or even worse sometimes so they're not the worst person on the planet. They start to say to themselves, 'This is human, I am human, others are human.'"

Gaining some perspective on their situations, and feeling supported by others, is a critically important threshold for people to cross as they start to seriously consider seeking treatment from a physician or psycho-therapist. And exchanging shame for hope is the most gratifying, if difficult, transformation an anxiety disorder patient can ever achieve, as he or she picks up the phone and steps firmly on the road to recovery.

Understanding Anxiety Disorders

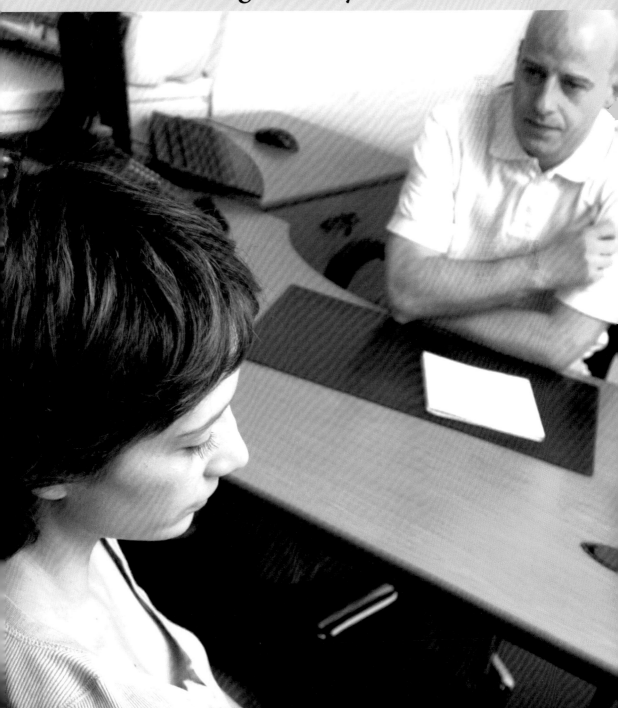

Defining Anxiety Disorders

Rebecca J. Frey and Teresa G. Odle

This excerpt from *The Gale Encyclopedia of Medicine* presents a general overview of anxiety disorders. Authors Rebecca J. Frey and Teresa G. Odle define anxiety disorders and offer background on the evolving classification of anxiety disorders in the *Diagnostic and Statistical Manual of Mental Disorders (DSM)*. The authors list the seven different groups of anxiety disorders and present several treatment options, including options that are derived from alternative sources. They conclude by presenting thoughts on recovery and prevention of symptoms by utilizing beneficial treatments. Frey is a medical writer from New Haven, Connecticut. Odle is a writer, editor, and member of the American Medical Writers Association.

The anxiety disorders are a group of mental disturbances characterized by anxiety as a central or core symptom. Although anxiety is a commonplace experience, not everyone who experiences it has an

Photo on previous page. Treatment options for anxiety disorders include psychotherapy and medication. (AJPhoto/ Photo Researchers, Inc.)

anxiety disorder. Anxiety is associated with a wide range of physical illnesses, medication side effects, and other psychiatric disorders.

The revisions of the *Diagnostic and Statistical Manual of Mental Disorders (DSM)* that took place after 1980 brought major changes in the classification of the anxiety disorders. Prior to 1980, psychiatrists classified patients on the basis of a theory that defined anxiety as the outcome of unconscious conflicts in the patient's mind. *DSM-III* (1980), *DSM-III-R* (1987), and *DSM-IV* (1994) introduced and refined a new classification that considered recent discoveries about the biochemical and posttraumatic origins of some types of anxiety. The present definitions are based on the external and reported symptom patterns of the disorders rather than on theories about their origins.

Anxiety disorders are the most common form of mental disturbance in the United States population. It is estimated that 28 million people suffer from an anxiety disorder every year. These disorders are a serious problem for the entire society because of their interference with patients' work, schooling, and family life. They also contribute to the high rates of alcohol and substance abuse in the United States. Anxiety disorders are an additional problem for health professionals because the physical symptoms of anxiety frequently bring people to primary care doctors or emergency rooms.

Seven Groups of Disorders

DSM-IV defines 12 types of anxiety disorders in the adult population. They can be grouped under seven headings:

- *Panic disorders with or without agoraphobia.* The chief characteristic of panic disorder is the occurrence of panic attacks coupled with fear of their recurrence. In clinical settings, agoraphobia is usually not a disorder by itself, but is typically associated with some form of panic disorder. Patients with agoraphobia are afraid of places or situations in which they might have a panic attack and be unable to leave or to find help. About 25% of patients with panic disorder develop obsessive-compulsive disorder (OCD).

- *Phobias.* These include specific phobias and social phobia. A phobia is an intense irrational fear of a specific object or situation that compels the patient to avoid it. Some phobias concern activities or objects that involve some risk (for example, flying or driving) but many are focused on harmless animals or other objects. Social phobia involves a fear of being humiliated, judged, or scrutinized. It manifests itself as a fear of performing certain functions in the presence of others, such as public speaking or using public lavatories.

A phobia is an irrational fear of a specific situation or an object, such as a needle. (Adam Gault/ Photo Researchers, Inc.)

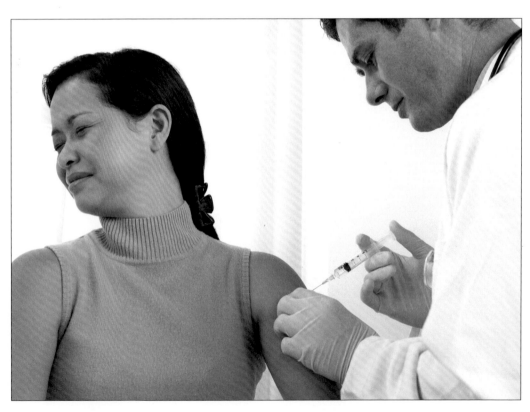

- *Obsessive-compulsive disorder (OCD).* This disorder is marked by unwanted, intrusive, persistent thoughts or repetitive behaviors that reflect the patient's anxiety or attempts to control it. It affects between 2–3% of the population and is much more common than was previously thought.
- *Stress disorders.* These include post-traumatic stress disorder (PTSD) and acute stress disorder. Stress disorders are symptomatic reactions to traumatic events in the patient's life.
- *Generalized anxiety disorder (GAD).* GAD is the most commonly diagnosed anxiety disorder and occurs most frequently in young adults.
- *Anxiety disorders due to known physical causes.* These include general medical conditions or substance abuse.
- *Anxiety disorder not otherwise specified.* This last category is not a separate type of disorder, but is included to cover symptoms that do not meet the specific *DSM-IV* criteria for other anxiety disorders.

Distribution of Disorders

All *DSM-IV* anxiety disorder diagnoses include a criterion of severity. The anxiety must be severe enough to interfere significantly with the patient's occupational or educational functioning, social activities or close relationships, and other customary activities.

The anxiety disorders vary widely in their frequency of occurrence in the general population, age of onset, family patterns, and gender distribution. The stress disorders and anxiety disorders caused by medical conditions or substance abuse are less age- and gender-specific. Whereas OCD affects males and females equally, GAD, panic disorder, and specific phobias all affect women more frequently than men. GAD and panic disorders are more likely to develop in young adults, while phobias and OCD can begin in childhood.

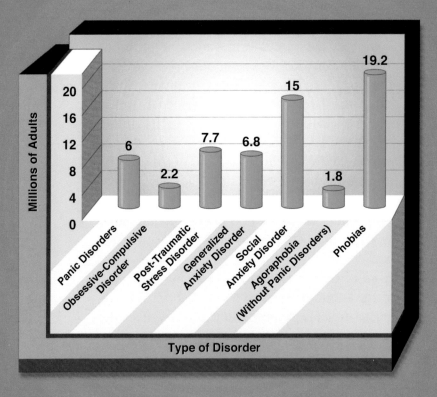

Number of American Adults with Anxiety Disorders

Millions of Adults

Panic Disorders	6
Obsessive-Compulsive Disorder	2.2
Post-Traumatic Stress Disorder	7.7
Generalized Anxiety Disorder	6.8
Social Anxiety Disorder	15
Agoraphobia (Without Panic Disorders)	1.8
Phobias	19.2

Type of Disorder

Taken from: National Institute of Mental Health.

DSM-IV defines one anxiety disorder as specific to children, namely, separation anxiety disorder. This disorder is defined as anxiety regarding separation from home or family that is excessive or inappropriate for the child's age. In some children, separation anxiety takes the form of school avoidance.

Children and adolescents can also be diagnosed with panic disorder, phobias, generalized anxiety disorder, and the post-traumatic stress syndromes.

The causes of anxiety include a variety of individual and general social factors, and may produce physical, cognitive, emotional, or behavioral symptoms. The patient's ethnic or cultural background may also influence his or her vulnerability to certain forms of anxiety. Genetic factors that lead to biochemical abnormalities may also play a role.

Anxiety in children may be caused by suffering from abuse, as well as by the factors that cause anxiety in adults.

Making a Diagnosis

The diagnosis of anxiety disorders is complicated by the variety of causes of anxiety and the range of disorders that may include anxiety as a symptom. Many patients who suffer from anxiety disorders have features or symptoms of more than one disorder. Patients whose anxiety is accounted for by another psychic disorder, such as schizophrenia or major depression, are not diagnosed with an anxiety disorder. A doctor examining an anxious patient will usually begin by ruling out diseases that are known to cause anxiety and then proceed to take the patient's medication history, in order to exclude side effects of prescription drugs. Most doctors will ask about caffeine consumption to see if the patient's dietary habits are a factor. The patient's work and family situation will also be discussed. Often, primary care physicians will exhaust resources looking for medical causes for general patient complaints which may indicate a physical illness. In 2004, the Anxiety Disorders Association of American published guidelines to better aid physicians in diagnosing and managing generalized anxiety disorder. Laboratory tests for blood sugar and thyroid function are also common.

There are no laboratory tests that can diagnose anxiety, although the doctor may order some specific tests to rule out disease conditions. Although there is no psychiatric test that can provide definite diagnoses of anxiety disorders, there are several short-answer interviews or symptom inventories that doctors can use to evaluate the intensity of a patient's anxiety and some of its associated features. These measures include the Hamilton Anxiety Scale and the Anxiety Disorders Interview Schedule (ADIS).

Treatment Options

For relatively mild anxiety disorders, psychotherapy alone may suffice. In general, doctors prefer to use a combination of medications and psychotherapy with more severely anxious patients. Most patients respond better to a combination of treatment methods than to either medications or psychotherapy in isolation. Because of the variety of medications and treatment approaches that are used to treat anxiety disorders, the doctor cannot predict in advance which combination will be most helpful to a specific patient. In many cases the doctor will need to try a new medication or treatment over a six- to eight-week period in order to assess its effectiveness. Treatment trials do not necessarily mean that the patient cannot be helped or that the doctor is incompetent.

Although anxiety disorders are not always easy to diagnose, there are several reasons why it is important for patients with severe anxiety symptoms to get help. Anxiety doesn't always go away by itself; it often progresses to panic attacks, phobias, and episodes of depression. Untreated anxiety disorders may eventually lead to a diagnosis of major depression, or interfere with the patient's education or ability to keep a job. It addition, many anxious patients develop addictions to drugs or alcohol when they try to "medicate" their symptoms. Moreover, since children learn ways of coping with anxiety from their parents, adults who get help for anxiety disorders are in a better position to help their families cope with factors that lead to anxiety than those who remain untreated.

Alternative treatments for anxiety cover a variety of approaches. Meditation and mindfulness training are thought beneficial to patients with phobias and panic disorder. Hydrotherapy is useful to some anxious patients because it promotes general relaxation of the nervous system. Yoga, aikido, t'ai chi, and dance therapy help patients work with the physical, as well as the emotional, tensions that either promote anxiety or are created by the anxiety.

Homeopathy and traditional Chinese medicine approach anxiety as a symptom of a systemic disorder. Homeopathic practitioners select a remedy based on other associated symptoms and the patient's general constitution. Chinese medicine regards anxiety as a blockage of *qi*, or vital force, inside the patient's body that is most likely to affect the lung and large intestine meridian flow. The practitioner of Chinese medicine chooses acupuncture point locations and/or herbal therapy to move the qi and rebalance the entire system in relation to the lung and large intestine.

> **FAST FACT**
>
> According to the Anxiety Disorders Association of America, anxiety disorders are the most common mental illness in the United States, affecting 40 million adults aged eighteen and older.

Recovery and Prevention

The prognosis for recovery depends on the specific disorder, the severity of the patient's symptoms, the specific causes of the anxiety, and the patient's degree of control over these causes.

Anxiety is an unavoidable feature of human existence. However, humans have some power over their reactions to anxiety-provoking events and situations. Cognitive therapy and meditation or mindfulness training appear to be beneficial in helping people lower their long-term anxiety levels.

Treating Anxiety Disorders

National Institute of Mental Health

This excerpt, from a booklet published by the National Institute of Mental Health, focuses on treatment options for anxiety disorders. The best treatment approach for most patients is some combination of medication and therapy. Medication will not cure an anxiety disorder, but it can help control symptoms. Among these medications are antidepressants, antianxiety drugs, and even beta blockers, which are traditionally used for heart conditions but have been successful at treating patients diagnosed with social phobia. Psychotherapy is another option for treatment and includes both cognitive-behavioral therapy and exposure-based therapy. Cognitive-behavioral therapy is used to help patients change how they think about their fears and how they react to those fears. Exposure-based therapy is used to treat phobias by slowly introducing the feared object or situation to the patient in an attempt to help them overcome their phobic behavior.

In general, anxiety disorders are treated with medication, specific types of psychotherapy, or both. Treatment choices depend on the problem and the per-

SOURCE: *Anxiety Disorders: National Institute of Mental Health.* Bethesda, MD: U.S. Department of Health and Human Services, 2009. Reproduced by permission.

son's preference. Before treatment begins, a doctor must conduct a careful diagnostic evaluation to determine whether a person's symptoms are caused by an anxiety disorder or a physical problem. If an anxiety disorder is diagnosed, the type of disorder or the combination of disorders that are present must be identified, as well as any coexisting conditions, such as depression or substance abuse. Sometimes alcoholism, depression, or other coexisting conditions have such a strong effect on the individual that treating the anxiety disorder must wait until the coexisting conditions are brought under control.

Treating Anxiety Disorders

Have you participated in any of the following to help manage your anxiety disorder?

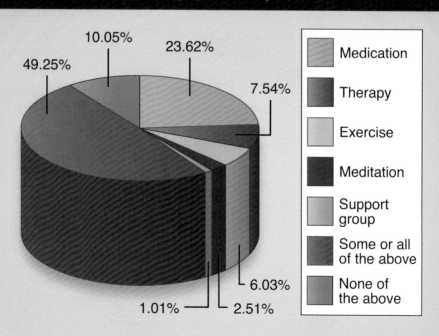

- Medication
- Therapy
- Exercise
- Meditation
- Support group
- Some or all of the above
- None of the above

49.25% 10.05% 23.62% 7.54% 1.01% 2.51% 6.03%

Taken from: Anxiety Disorders Association of America.

People with anxiety disorders who have already received treatment should tell their current doctor about that treatment in detail. If they received medication, they should tell their doctor what medication was used, what the dosage was at the beginning of treatment, whether the dosage was increased or decreased while they were under treatment, what side effects occurred, and whether the treatment helped them become less anxious. If they received psychotherapy, they should describe the type of therapy, how often they attended sessions, and whether the therapy was useful.

Often people believe that they have "failed" at treatment or that the treatment didn't work for them when, in fact, it was not given for an adequate length of time or was administered incorrectly. Sometimes people must try several different treatments or combinations of treatment before they find the one that works for them.

Medication will not cure anxiety disorders, but it can keep them under control while the person receives psychotherapy. Medication must be prescribed by physicians, usually psychiatrists, who can either offer psychotherapy themselves or work as a team with psychologists, social workers, or counselors who provide psychotherapy. The principal medications used for anxiety disorders are antidepressants, anti-anxiety drugs, and beta-blockers to control some of the physical symptoms. With proper treatment, many people with anxiety disorders can lead normal, fulfilling lives.

Antidepressant Options

Antidepressants were developed to treat depression but are also effective for anxiety disorders. Although these medications begin to alter brain chemistry after the very first dose, their full effect requires a series of changes to occur; it is usually about 4 to 6 weeks before symptoms start to fade. It is important to continue taking these medications long enough to let them work.

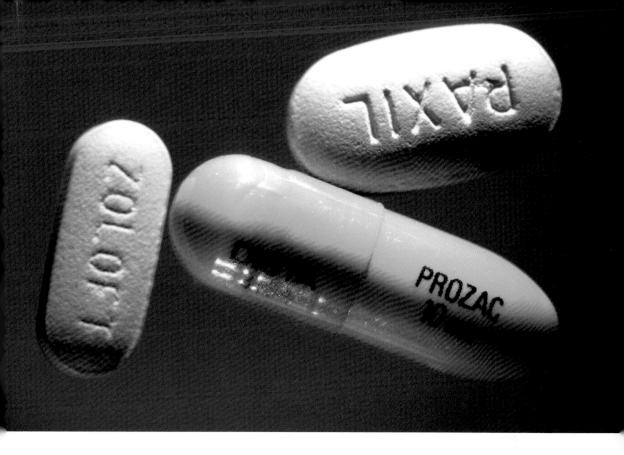

Some of the newest antidepressants are called selective serotonin reuptake inhibitors, or SSRIs. SSRIs alter the levels of the neurotransmitter serotonin in the brain, which, like other neurotransmitters, helps brain cells communicate with one another.

Fluoxetine (Prozac®), sertraline (Zoloft®), escitalopram (Lexapro®), paroxetine (Paxil®), and citalopram (Celexa®) are some of the SSRIs commonly prescribed for panic disorder, OCD [obsessive-compulsive disorder], PTSD [post-traumatic stress disorder], and social phobia. SSRIs are also used to treat panic disorder when it occurs in combination with OCD, social phobia, or depression. Venlafaxine (Effexor®), a drug closely related to the SSRIs, is used to treat GAD [generalized anxiety disorder]. These medications are started at low doses and gradually increased until they have a beneficial effect.

SSRIs have fewer side effects than older antidepressants, but they sometimes produce slight nausea or jitters

Some of the newest antidepressants are the selective serotonin reuptake inhibitors (SSRIs), which include Zoloft, Prozac, and Paxil. (Leonard Kesseb, FBPA/ Photo Researchers, Inc.)

when people first start to take them. These symptoms fade with time. Some people also experience sexual dysfunction with SSRIs, which may be helped by adjusting the dosage or switching to another SSRI.

Tricyclics are older than SSRIs and work as well as SSRIs for anxiety disorders other than OCD. They are also started at low doses that are gradually increased. They sometimes cause dizziness, drowsiness, dry mouth, and weight gain, which can usually be corrected by changing the dosage or switching to another tricyclic medication.

Tricyclics include imipramine (Tofranil®), which is prescribed for panic disorder and GAD, and clomipramine (Anafranil®), which is the only tricyclic antidepressant useful for treating OCD.

Monoamine oxidase inhibitors (MAOIs) are the oldest class of antidepressant medications. The MAOIs most commonly prescribed for anxiety disorders are phenelzine (Nardil®), followed by tranylcypromine (Parnate®), and isocarboxazid (Marplan®), which are useful in treating panic disorder and social phobia. People who take MAOIs cannot eat a variety of foods and beverages (including cheese and red wine) that contain tyramine or take certain medications, including some types of birth control pills, pain relievers (such as Advil®, Motrin®, or Tylenol®), cold and allergy medications, and herbal supplements; these substances can interact with MAOIs to cause dangerous increases in blood pressure. The development of a new MAOI skin patch may help lessen these risks. MAOIs can also react with SSRIs to produce a serious condition called "serotonin syndrome," which can cause confusion, hallucinations, increased sweating, muscle stiffness, seizures, changes in blood pressure or heart rhythm, and other potentially life-threatening conditions.

FAST FACT

Only one-third of people who experience symptoms related to anxiety disorders actually visit a doctor.

Anti-anxiety Drugs

High-potency benzodiazepines combat anxiety and have few side effects other than drowsiness. Because people can get used to them and may need higher and higher doses to get the same effect, benzodiazepines are generally prescribed for short periods of time, especially for people who have abused drugs or alcohol and who become dependent on medication easily. One exception to this rule is people with panic disorder, who can take benzodiazepines for up to a year without harm.

Clonazepam (Klonopin®) is used for social phobia and GAD, lorazepam (Ativan®) is helpful for panic disorder, and alprazolam (Xanax®) is useful for both panic disorder and GAD.

Some people experience withdrawal symptoms if they stop taking benzodiazepines abruptly instead of tapering off, and anxiety can return once the medication is stopped. These potential problems have led some physicians to shy away from using these drugs or to use them in inadequate doses.

Buspirone (Buspar®), an azapirone, is a newer anti-anxiety medication used to treat GAD. Possible side effects include dizziness, headaches, and nausea. Unlike benzodiazepines, buspirone must be taken consistently for at least 2 weeks to achieve an anti-anxiety effect.

Beta-blockers, such as propranolol (Inderal®), which is used to treat heart conditions, can prevent the physical symptoms that accompany certain anxiety disorders, particularly social phobia. When a feared situation can be predicted (such as giving a speech), a doctor may prescribe a beta-blocker to keep physical symptoms of anxiety under control.

Cognitive-Behavioral Therapy

Psychotherapy involves talking with a trained mental health professional, such as a psychiatrist, psychologist, social worker, or counselor, to discover what caused an anxiety disorder and how to deal with its symptoms.

Cognitive-behavioral therapy (CBT) is very useful in treating anxiety disorders. The cognitive part helps people change the thinking patterns that support their fears, and the behavioral part helps people change the way they react to anxiety-provoking situations.

For example, CBT can help people with panic disorder learn that their panic attacks are not really heart attacks and help people with social phobia learn how to overcome the belief that others are always watching and judging them. When people are ready to confront their fears, they are shown how to use exposure techniques to desensitize themselves to situations that trigger their anxieties. People with OCD who fear dirt and germs are encouraged to get their hands dirty and wait increasing amounts of time before washing them. The therapist helps the person cope with the anxiety that waiting produces; after the exercise has been repeated a number of times, the anxiety diminishes. People with social phobia may be encouraged to spend time in feared social situations without giving in to the temptation to flee and to make small social blunders and observe how people respond to them. Since the response is usually far less harsh than the person fears, these anxieties are lessened. People with PTSD may be supported through recalling their traumatic event in a safe situation, which helps reduce the fear it produces. CBT therapists also teach deep breathing and other types of exercises to relieve anxiety and encourage relaxation.

Exposure-Based Behavioral Therapy

Exposure-based behavioral therapy has been used for many years to treat specific phobias. The person gradually encounters the object or situation that is feared, perhaps at first only through pictures or tapes, then later face-to-face. Often the therapist will accompany the person to a feared situation to provide support and guidance.

CBT is undertaken when people decide they are ready for it and with their permission and cooperation. To be effective, the therapy must be directed at the person's specific anxieties and must be tailored to his or her needs. There are no side effects other than the discomfort of temporarily increased anxiety.

CBT or behavioral therapy often lasts about 12 weeks. It may be conducted individually or with a group of people who have similar problems. Group therapy is particularly effective for social phobia. Often "homework" is assigned for participants to complete between sessions. There is some evidence that the benefits of CBT last longer than those of medication for people with panic disorder, and the same may be true for OCD, PTSD, and social phobia. If a disorder recurs at a later date, the same therapy can be used to treat it successfully a second time.

Medication can be combined with psychotherapy for specific anxiety disorders, and this is the best treatment approach for many people.

Anxiety and Depression Are Closely Related

Michael L. Nichols

This article explores the relationship between anxiety disorders and clinical depression and cites recent studies demonstrating a closer linkage between the two than was previously believed. The author, Michael L. Nichols, contends that not only do patients with anxiety disorders and depression share similar coping strategies and genetic traits, but that they benefit from similar treatment options, such as cognitive-behavioral therapy and medication. Nichols concludes by speculating about a possible reclassification of the two disorders into a broader spectrum disorder in the *Diagnostic and Statistical Manual of Mental Disorders*, the American Psychiatric Association's authoritative book of diagnoses for physicians and therapists.

Nichols runs the Anxiety, Panic & Health Web site, which provides information and research for those who suffer from, or want to learn more about, anxiety disorders. A husband and father, Nichols has personal experience in dealing with an anxiety disorder and started his Web site with the hope that he could help others better cope and understand their affliction.

Modern psychiatry has long held that Anxiety Disorder and depression are two distinct conditions.

However, in the real world, many suffer from both. Surveys show that half of Anxiety Disorder sufferers also have symptoms of clinical depression. And 60–70 percent of people with major depression also have an Anxiety Disorder. Evidence is growing that they are really two aspects of one disorder. Looking at them that way, some experts say, could speed the development of therapy and medications that better treat both conditions.

David Barlow, director of the Center for Anxiety and Related Disorders at Boston University, states that:

> [Anxiety Disorders and depression are] probably two sides of the same coin. The genetics seem to be the same; the neurobiology seems to overlap.

This [article] explores several similarities between Anxiety Disorders and depression, along with the risks of getting both disorders, the benefits of early treatment, and a summary of how the disorders are treated together.

Reactions to Anxiety and Depression

Anxiety Disorders and depression feed on each other, each making the other worse. David Barlow says that, "Some people with the vulnerability react with anxiety to life stressors and some, in addition, go beyond that to become depressed." He adds,

> Depression seems to be a shutdown. Anxiety is a kind of looking to the future, seeing dangerous things that might happen in the next hour, day or weeks. Depression is all that with the addition of "I really don't think I'm going to be able to cope with this, maybe I'll just give up." It's shutdown marked by mental, cognitive or behavioral slowing.

Most people who suffer from depression or anxiety disorders share the common trait of avoidant behavior. (**LADA**/**Photo Researchers, Inc.**)

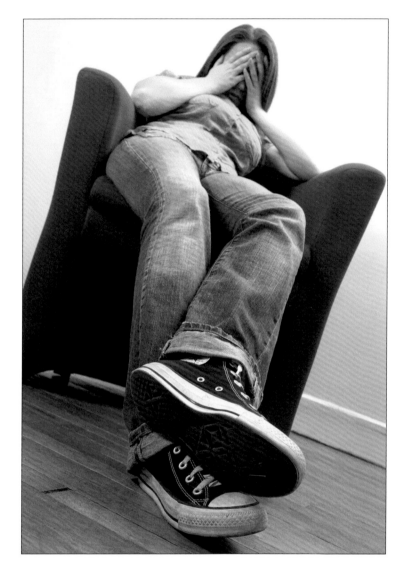

In groundbreaking research, Kenneth S. Kendler, a behavioral geneticist from Virginia Commonwealth University in Richmond, offers a new way of looking at psychiatric conditions. He sees a small cluster of genetic risk factors creating "internalizing disorders" such as Anxiety Disorder and depression, which cause sufferers to be miserable. Another set of genetic factors finds expression in "externalizing disorders" such as substance abuse and antisocial behavior—conditions that make others around them miserable.

Anxiety Disorders and depression share an avoidant coping style. Sufferers avoid what they fear instead of developing the skills to handle the kinds of situations that make them uncomfortable. Often, a lack of social skills is at the root of their avoidant behavior. Jerilyn Ross, LICSW [Licensed Independent Clinical Social Worker and] president of the Anxiety Disorders Association of America [ADAA], says,

> [The link between Social Phobia and depression is] dramatic. It often affects young people who can't go out, can't date, don't have friends. They're very isolated, all alone, and feel cut off.

Shared Genetics

At the center of the double disorder are shared brain mechanisms gone awry. Studies have shown that the stress response system is overactive in patients with both Anxiety Disorders and depression, which sends the emotional centers of the brain—including the "fear center" in the amygdala—into hyperactivity. Secretions of the stress hormone cortisol, triggered by repeated trauma, reduce the activity of the gene that produces the 5-HT1A serotonin receptor, which is an important brain messenger implicated in both Anxiety Disorders and depression.

Another study from researchers at the National Institute of Mental Health has found that, in people with both Panic Disorder and depression, there is a significant decrease in a type of receptor (5-HT1A) for the neurotransmitter serotonin.

Early Treatment

Anxiety usually precedes depression developmentally, with Anxiety Disorders most commonly beginning in late childhood or adolescence and depression a few years later, in the mid-20s. Psychologist Michael Yapko of San Diego points out a flaw in thinking common in both disorders:

> The shared cornerstone of Anxiety and depression is the perceptual process of overestimating the risk in a situation and underestimating personal resources for coping.

Yapko sees a huge opportunity for the prevention of depression, as the average age of first onset is now mid-20s. He says,

> A young person is not likely to outgrow anxiety unless treated and taught cognitive skills. But aggressive treatment of the anxiety when it appears can prevent the subsequent development of depression.

Who Is at Risk?

There's definitely a family heredity component in the risk for developing Anxiety Disorder and depression together. Joseph Himle, Ph.D., Associate Director of the Anxiety Disorders Unit at the University of Michigan, says,

> Looking at [what disorders populate] the family history of a person who presents with either primary Anxiety or depression provides a clue to whether he or she will end up with both.

The nature of the Anxiety Disorder also has an influence. Obsessive-Compulsive Disorder, Panic Disorder and Social Phobia are particularly associated with depression. Specific Phobias are less so.

Age plays a role, as well. Himle states,

> A person who develops an Anxiety Disorder for the first time after age 40 is likely also to have depression. Someone who develops panic attacks for the first time at age 50 often has a history of depression or is experiencing depression at the same time.

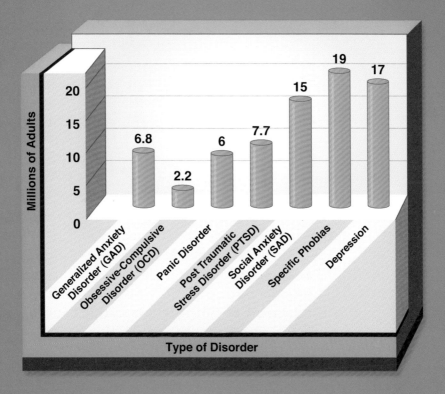

U.S. Adults Affected by Anxiety Disorders and Depression

Taken from: Anxiety Disorders Association of America, www.adaa.org/AboutADAA/PressRoom/Stats&Facts.asp/ www.wrongdiagnosis.com/d/depression/stats.htm.

Sometimes a vulnerability to Anxiety Disorders are inherited by a person, and sometimes they are transmitted to children by parental overconcern. Yapko states that:

The largest group of depression/Anxiety sufferers is Baby Boomers. The fastest growing group is their children. They can't teach kids what they don't know. Plus their desire to raise perfect children puts tremendous pressures on the kids. They're creating a bumper crop of anxious/depressed children.

Similar Treatments for Anxiety and Depression

The treatments that work best for depression also combat Anxiety Disorder. Cognitive-Behavioral Therapy (CBT) is very successful in working with the response patterns central to both conditions. And the drugs most commonly used against depression, the SSRI's, or selective serotonin reuptake inhibitors, have also been proved effective against an array of Anxiety Disorders, from Social Phobia to Panic Disorder and Post Traumatic Stress Disorder (PTSD). Which drug a patient should get is based more on what can be tolerated rather than on symptoms.

Treatment rarely centers on which disorder, the Anxiety Disorder or the depression, came first. "In many cases," says Ross of the ADAA, "the depression exists because the anxiety is so draining. Once you treat the anxiety, the depression lifts."

Treatment usually is targeted at depression and the Anxiety Disorder simultaneously. Himle states,

> There's increasing interest in treating both disorders at the same time. Cognitive Behavioral Therapy is particularly attractive because it has applications to both.

But sometimes the depression is so incapacitating that it has to be overcome first. For example, depression often interferes with exposure therapy for Anxiety, in which people gradually confront situations they avoid because they give rise to overwhelming fear. Himle notes:

> Exposure therapy requires substantial effort. That's effort that depressed people often do not have available to them.

Road to Recovery

Antidepressants can make a difference with both Anxiety Disorders and depression. Many SSRIs are approved for use in Anxiety Disorders and are the first line of drug therapy. But which drug works best for whom cannot be predicted in advance; it may take some trial and error.

Ross finds CBT 80-90 percent successful in getting people functioning well, "provided it's done correctly." Not all psychotherapy is CBT, which has a very specific set of procedures, nor is every mental health professional trained in CBT. "Patients have to make sure that is what they are really getting."

Treatment averages 12 to 15 weeks, and patients can expect to see significant improvement by six weeks. Ross says,

> CBT doesn't involve years and years of talk therapy. There's homework, practice and development of lifestyle changes. Once patients learn how to identify the trigger thoughts or feelings, or events or people, they need to keep doing that. CBT gives people the tools they need.

Medication and CBT are equally effective in reducing Anxiety Disorders and depression. But CBT is better at preventing relapse, and it creates greater patient satisfaction. "It's more empowering," says Yapko. "Patients like feeling responsible for their own success." Further, new data suggests that the active coping CBT encourages creates new brain circuits that circumvent the dysfunctional response pathways.

Future Classifications

The strong separation of Anxiety Disorders and depression into two disorders was introduced [by] the third (1980) and fourth (1994) editions of the *Diagnostic and Statistical Manual of Mental Disorders (DSM)* of the American Psychiatric Association.

FAST FACT

The Healthy Place Web site reports that in one study, 85 percent of those with major depression were also diagnosed with generalized anxiety disorder while 35 percent had symptoms of a panic disorder.

The *DSM* is not only used for diagnoses of mental illnesses worldwide, it shapes the mindset of mental health professionals formulating treatments for Anxiety Disorder and depression. With the increasing realization that Anxiety Disorders and depression are closely related, better psychotherapy strategies are being developed to deal with both disorders simultaneously. With all the research being done on the interconnectedness of Anxiety Disorders and depression, it will be interesting to see how these disorders are handled in the new edition of the *DSM*, due in 2012. It may very well be that the diagnoses of two decades will be set on their ears by this new information.

In a recent article published in the *British Medical Journal,* physicians Edward Shorter of Canada and Peter Tyrer of England contend that this separation of Anxiety Disorder and depression, along with several different varieties of Anxiety, is a "wrong classification" that has led the pharmaceutical industry down a "blind alley." It is also "one reason for the big slowdown in drug discovery in psychiatric drugs," they say, adding that it is difficult to create effective drugs for marketing-driven disease "niches."

Managing Obsessive-Compulsive Disorder

Mark Rowh

In this article, Mark Rowh focuses on obsessive-compulsive disorder (OCD), an anxiety disorder that affects as many as one in two hundred kids and teens. Rowh explains the disease and the symptoms associated with it, such as repeatedly checking that the door is locked or excessively brushing teeth. Though the reason for the disease is still unclear, it is a brain-based disorder. Rowh contends that help is available and the ultimate goal is to control the disease and its symptoms. Rowh is a professional educator and widely published author. He is the author of Great Jobs for Chemistry Majors *and other books.*

As Amanda Lazaro entered her teen years, she found herself worrying all the time, especially about germs. She avoided crowds and washed her hands over and over until they bled. She also hid her worries from others.

SOURCE: Mark Rowh, "The ABC's of OCD: Teens Who Have Obsessive-Compulsive Disorder Need Not Suffer in Silence," *Current Health 2*, April/May 2007, p. 23. Copyright © 2007 Weekly Reader Corp. Reproduced by permission.

"I would constantly hide [my behavior], and if it was brought to my attention, I would laugh it off," says Lazaro, who's now 22 and living in Boston. "But when I found myself not being able to go out with friends because there was a chance that I could bring home a disease, it became very hard to hide and more of a problem." Although she didn't realize it at first, Lazaro's feelings were symptoms of obsessive-compulsive disorder (OCD).

A Common Problem and Its Sufferers

Experiences like Lazaro's are not as unusual as you might think. As many as one in every 200 kids and teens has OCD, according to the American Academy of Child and Adolescent Psychiatry. And at least one-third of all adults with OCD began dealing with it in childhood.

People who have this disorder typically suffer from both obsessions (persistent thoughts or ideas that are intrusive or excessive) and compulsions (acts or behaviors done repeatedly). For reasons that may not make sense to others, OCD sufferers feel the need to perform certain rituals. They might count objects, check repeatedly that a door is locked, brush teeth excessively, or repeat other behaviors.

In some cases, the connection between obsessions and compulsions may seem obvious. For example, someone with an overriding fear of getting sick may wash his or her hands dozens of times a day to get rid of germs. But someone else might stomp his or her feet or repeatedly count strings of numbers as an indirect way of coping with obsessive fears or anxieties.

"Everyone worries sometimes," explains Dr. Eve Wood, a psychiatrist at the University of Arizona. "But people with OCD have brains that get stuck on particular thoughts and behaviors."

Just why this happens is not entirely clear, but the disorder has its origins in the human brain. Scientists have learned that the front area of the brain, where errors are

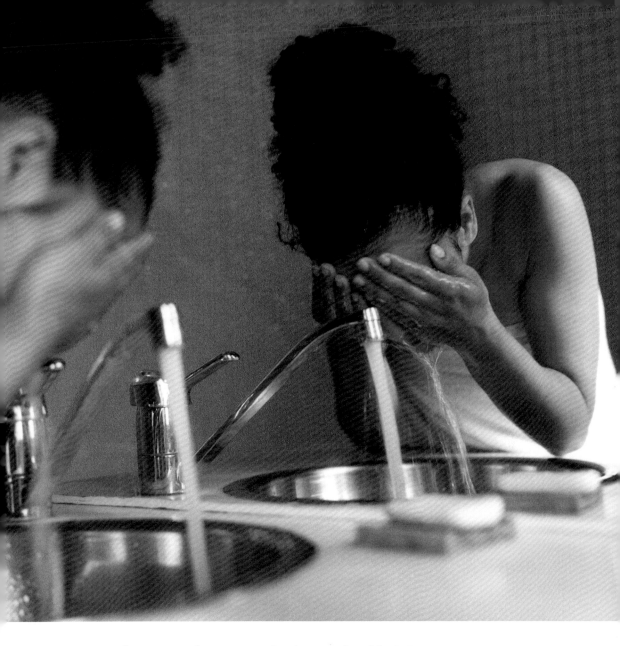

processed, seems to be more active in people with OCD. The recent discovery of an "OCD gene" may mean that OCD can be inherited in some families. But more often than not, heredity doesn't seem to be a factor, and the root causes of the disorder are still unknown.

A common trait of obsessive compulsive disorder is an obsession with cleanliness. (Cristina Pderazzini/Photo Researchers, Inc.)

D'Arcy Lyness, a Pennsylvania psychologist and an editor at TeensHealth.org, says that with OCD, it's as if the brain's anxiety "alarm system" is on overdrive. "OCD creates a terrible sense of uncertainty, doubt, worry, or fear in a person's mind," she says. "People with OCD have upsetting or scary thoughts or images and can't shake them. They feel drawn into doing compulsions to get relief from the bad thoughts and feelings."

Hiding the Obsessions

Too often, the stress of OCD is compounded by concerns about what others might think. "Lots of teens . . . hide the symptoms of the disorder," says Mona Berman, a psychotherapist based in Northfield, Ill. "They think they are weird and are embarrassed." Such fears

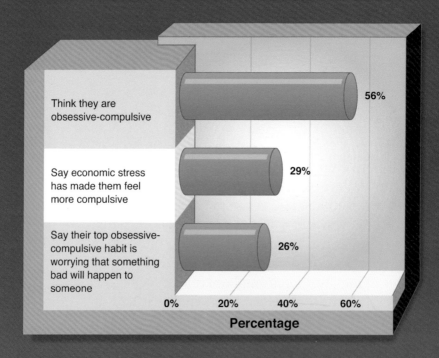

Poll Respondents Express Opinions on Obsessive-Compulsive Disorder

Think they are obsessive-compulsive — 56%

Say economic stress has made them feel more compulsive — 29%

Say their top obsessive-compulsive habit is worrying that something bad will happen to someone — 26%

Taken from: *Health*, "Health.com poll," April 2009, p. 141.

are frequently unfounded, and teens with OCD may be surprised to find that others are more understanding than they anticipated. But the fear of being teased or laughed at can be very real.

Nevertheless, the diagnosis of OCD can be something of a relief. That was the case for Scott, a 13-year-old from Chicago. He found himself worrying that something was wrong with his food, and during meals he spent a lot of time picking out bits he thought might be contaminated. He also developed habits such as pulling at his lip, tugging his hair, and [washing] his hands for an unusually long time.

"I often felt very anxious, and worried constantly about things like getting sick and missing school," he says. "And I tried to hide these things." But when his parents took him to a therapist who pointed out that Scott had OCD, he was relieved to learn that his problems were not all that unusual and that he was not alone. The attitudes of his friends also helped. "They've been really cool about it," he says. "Nobody has made fun of me."

Managing OCD

Fortunately, plenty of help is available for anyone with OCD. Over the long term, experts usually speak in terms of controlling rather than totally curing it. But the problems caused by the disorder can be surmounted. "OCD is a highly treatable condition," says Stephen Hinshaw of the psychology department at the University of California, Berkeley. "Medications are quite effective." Most of the medicines used, known as selective serotonin-reuptake inhibitors, work by affecting a chemical messenger in the brain called serotonin. "Cognitive-behavioral therapy is also very helpful," Hinshaw adds. This type of therapy focuses on replacing distorted thoughts and finding ways to modify compulsive behavior.

Certainly, teens who suspect they might have OCD should seek help. A good first step is to confide in a parent. Family doctors, school counselors, and therapists can provide help in controlling the disorder.

It's also important to avoid jumping to conclusions. If you have anxieties or spend a lot of time being neat and clean, that doesn't necessarily mean you have OCD. But if you find yourself getting "stuck" on certain rituals or have overriding concerns that just won't go away, you might want to talk with a parent, a physician, or a mental health professional.

Living with OCD

Once they get help, most people who have OCD learn to deal with it. "I feel a lot better now," says Scott, who continues to see a therapist and take medicine for OCD. "I still get anxious sometimes, but I've learned this is a part of me, and I can live with it."

Lazaro has had a similar experience. The challenges of OCD have not gone away completely, but she has learned to cope with them. Lazaro uses meditation and yoga to diminish worries and frame more positive thoughts. "My OCD is less of a problem in my life now," she says. "I still wash my hands constantly and find myself freaking out when someone moves my picture frame from its appropriate placement, but I am able to go out and touch a doorknob in public and then wait until I get home to wash my hands."

At the moment, Lazaro's biggest concern is coping when people cough or sneeze. She finds grocery shopping during cold and flu season especially "unbearable" but is now able to handle touching a shopping cart. "OCD is a livable disorder," Lazaro concludes. "The challenge is finding a way to control the disorder so that it does not take over your life."

FAST FACT

According to the National Institute of Mental Health, about 2.3% of the United States population aged 18–54 has obsessive-compulsive disorder in a given year.

Common Obsessions and Compulsions

Obsessions (worries that won't go away)
- Undue fear of dirt, germs, or illness
- Overriding fear that something bad will happen to oneself or loved ones
- Obsessive need for neatness or order
- Focus on recurring words, sentences, songs, or numbers

Compulsions (behaviors done repeatedly)
- Excessive or repetitive hand washing
- Frequent arrangement or rearrangement of objects
- Excessive bathing or flossing or brushing of teeth
- Repeated checks that a door is locked
- Need to go in and out a door a certain number of times
- Counting, checking, repeating, and reviewing of tasks
- Tapping or stepping in a certain pattern

CHAPTER 2

Controversies Surrounding Anxiety Disorders

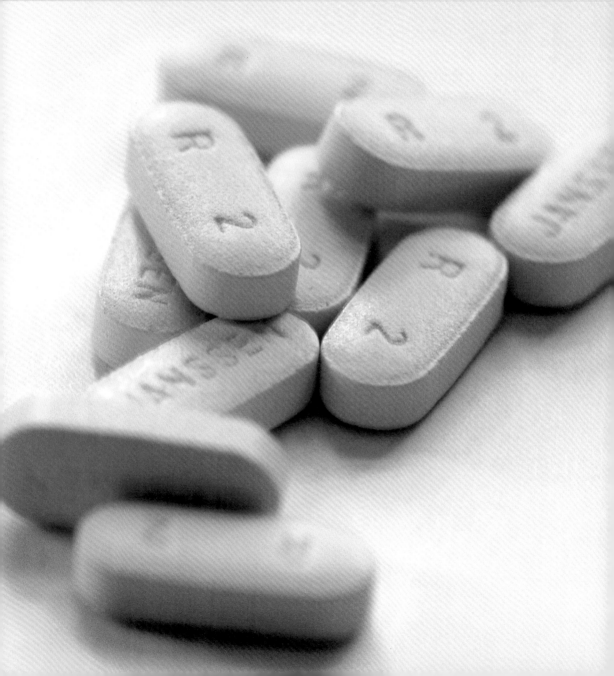

Anxiety Disorders Are Overdiagnosed and Overtreated

Philip Hickey

In this article posted on the Web site Behaviorism and Mental Health, Philip Hickey argues that the pharmaceutical industry, in conjunction with the nation's psychiatrists, have exploited people's tendency to look for easy solutions to difficult life problems. Instead of encouraging patients to understand the reasons for their stress and to make appropriate life changes, Hickey contends that psychiatrists too often diagnose the patient with an anxiety disorder and put them on medication that the pharmaceutical industry has heavily marketed for profit gain. Hickey believes that anxiety has an evolutionary basis that should serve as a warning sign for people to address their problems and that it should not be treated like a disorder by masking its symptoms with drugs.

Hickey is a licensed psychologist, presently retired. He has worked in clinical and managerial positions in the mental health, corrections, and addictions fields in the United States and England.

Photo on facing page. Some new drugs used to treat anxiety, such as Rispendal (pictured), are controversial. (Chris Gallagher/Photo Researchers, Inc.)

SOURCE: Philip Hickey, "Anxiety Disorders," BehaviorismandMental Health.com, April 7, 2009. Reproduced by permission.

Fear is the *normal* human response to imminent danger. It is an adaptive response, in that it is helpful to survival, and it occurs in almost all animal species. When our cave-dwelling ancestors were attacked by mountain lions, they probably experienced acute fear. This fear gave them an extra burst of energy to flee the danger, or, if flight were impossible, to turn and fight.

Today in most parts of the world, there is little danger of attack from wild animals. As areas develop economically and culturally, these kinds of acute dangers are systematically eliminated or at least drastically reduced. Close encounters with tornadoes, hurricanes, rattlesnakes, car accidents, etc., can still arouse full-blown fear responses, but most people in developed countries can go months—even years—without experiencing these kinds of situations.

The Marketing of Anxiety

Anxiety, however, is a different matter. Anxiety is essentially a fear response that doesn't quite take off. It is a constant feature of modern life. Just as industrial and commercial development entailed the systematic reduction of acute dangers, it involved an equally systematic *increase* in situations that provoke anxiety. Indeed, it could be argued that the production and maintenance of anxiety is an integral component of modern marketing.

The purpose of commercials is to generate within people feelings of insecurity and concern. The range of worries that are exploited in this way is limited only by the imaginations of the marketers. From all quarters we are bombarded with anxiety-producing messages, such as: you are not attractive; your television set is too small; your car is too old; your clothes are out of style; your hair is too gray (or oily, or dry); your libido is inadequate; your kitchen is outdated; your breasts are too small (female); your penis is too small (male); your computer is too old; your house needs to be painted; you have too

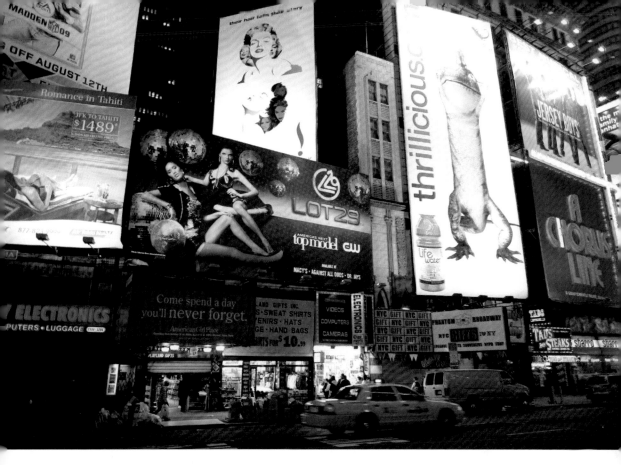

little hair on your head; you have too much hair everywhere else, etc., etc. . . . The purpose of these messages is to generate within us feelings of anxiety and insecurity so that we will buy more stuff. Of course the "fix" is only temporary, and the process continues pretty much from cradle to grave.

Advertisements that evoke feelings of fear or inadequacy can produce anxiety. (Kay Nietfeld/dpa/Landov)

From Biology to Malady

It is not being suggested that the marketers invented anxiety. Our ancestors in the caves probably experienced concern and anxiety if they heard unusual noises from outside the cave at night. This kind of anxiety is useful in that it increases vigilance and prepares the organism for a rapid response should this become necessary. In modern life there are many situations in which a certain amount of anxiety is appropriate and adaptive. On the highway, for instance, a sudden increase in the traffic density usually elicits a measure of anxiety. This anxiety sharpens our attention and helps us avoid mishaps. Similarly, most people will experience some anxiety if caught out in a severe storm, especially in tornado country. These are natural stressors and the anxiety they provoke is appropriate and helpful.

In addition, people who have had unpleasant experiences will likely feel some anxiety if exposed to similar circumstances later in life, and, in fact, will generally go to considerable pains to avoid such circumstances. People, for instance, who were teased and taunted during childhood will often in later life avoid situations where they might be exposed to criticism or ridicule.

What the marketers have done, however, is they have taken this natural adaptive mechanism and exploited it

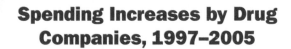

Spending Increases by Drug Companies, 1997–2005

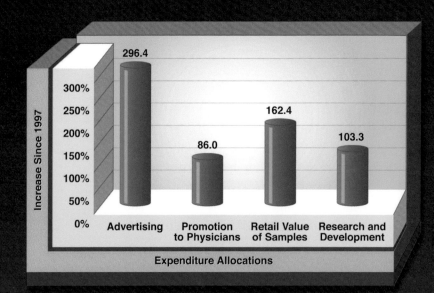

Taken from: U.S. Government Accountability Office.

endlessly for their own gain and to the detriment of the public. In this they have been extraordinarily successful, so that at present we experience worry and anxiety—not only with regards to genuine concerns—but also with regards to an enormous range of matters which are truly trivial and inconsequential. What used to be the land of the free and the home of the brave has degenerated into a nation of worriers and fretters. But the fundamental point is that anxiety, in and of itself, is normal—it is an integral part of our normal day-to-day existence, and serves a useful purpose. What the American Psychiatric Association and the pharmaceutical companies have done, however, is redefine anxiety as a pathology—an illness—that needs to be treated by taking pills.

List of Anxiety Disorders

The *DSM* [*Diagnostic and Statistical Manual of Mental Disorders*] lists the following anxiety disorders:
- Panic disorder without agoraphobia
- Panic disorder with agoraphobia
- Agoraphobia without panic disorder
- Specific phobia
- Social phobia
- Obsessive compulsive disorder
- Posttraumatic stress disorder
- Acute stress disorder
- Generalized anxiety disorder
- Anxiety disorder due to a general medical condition
- Substance induced anxiety disorder
- Separation anxiety disorder
- Sexual aversion disorder

And of course,

- Anxiety disorder not otherwise specified (n.o.s.)

The list is self-explanatory and is designed to cover as wide a range of anxiety-provoking situations as possible. The inclusion of the n.o.s. diagnosis at the end of the list ensures that anyone experiencing anxiety or worry concerning any matter whatsoever can be assigned a diagnosis and can enter the ranks of the "mentally ill." *DSM* specifies that for a diagnosis to be made, the anxiety has to "interfere with the person's functioning" or "cause marked distress." In practice, these qualifiers are sufficiently vague that virtually anyone can be given an anxiety diagnosis. People who go to counselors for help with stress or life choices are often assigned a diagnosis of Generalized Anxiety Disorder. They are "enrolled" in the ranks of the mentally ill, and their numbers swell the already inflated statistics. . . .

Real Reasons for Anxiety

Consider, for instance, a person who for several years has succumbed to the Madison Avenue [advertising] hype. This individual has bought a new house, a big car, an entertainment center, membership at an expensive country club, etc. Although apparently wealthy, he actually has no money in the bank and is completely dependent on his paycheck to remain solvent. He now receives information that his company is considering lay-offs, and he fears that his name may be on the list. Meanwhile, he discovers that his sixteen-year-old son is doing drugs, his fourteen-year-old daughter is sexually active, and his wife has been "seeing" someone else. Understandably, he is becoming somewhat anxious. In fact, he is beside himself with worry. He's not sleeping well. He's gone off his food, and he's beginning to make serious mistakes in his work. He doesn't actually see much of his family, but when he does, he finds himself being increasingly irritable and grouchy.

Although this is a purely hypothetical case, there are a great number of people in our society who are living variations of this kind of scenario—sometimes for years on end. Their lives have become untenable, and their anxiety and worry are entirely appropriate. Things are out of control. They *need* to be worried, and they need to be taking corrective action.

If our hypothetical worrier goes to a mental health practitioner, however, he will be given a diagnosis of Generalized Anxiety Disorder (an invented illness) and a prescription for anti-anxiety pills. He is given the false and destructive message that the problem is simply an illness—a chemical imbalance—and that taking the pills will correct the imbalance in the same way that insulin injections enable a diabetic to function normally. The notion that his life is out of control and that certain fundamental changes need to be made is seldom even addressed. . . .

Criteria for Diagnosis

The APA's [American Psychiatric Association's] criteria for a diagnosis of Generalized Anxiety Disorder are listed below:

A. Excessive anxiety and worry (apprehensive expectations), occurring more days than not for at least 6 months, about a number of events or activities (such as work or school performance).
B. The person finds it difficult to control the worry.
C. The anxiety and worry are associated with three (or more) of the following six symptoms (with at least some symptoms present for more days than not for the past 6 months). Note: Only one item is required in children.
   (1) restlessness or feeling keyed up or on edge
   (2) being easily fatigued
   (3) difficulty concentrating or mind going blank
   (4) irritability
   (5) muscle tension
   (6) sleep disturbance (difficulty falling or staying asleep, or restless unsatisfying sleep)
D. The focus of the anxiety and worry is not confined to features of [another mental disorder]

E. The anxiety, worry, or physical symptoms cause clinically significant distress or impairment in social, occupational, or other important areas of functioning.

F. The disturbance is not due to the direct physiological effects of a substance . . . or a general medical condition . . . or [another mental disorder].

The reader will readily appreciate that our hypothetical worrier described above, and the millions more in the same boat, are easily embraced within the above criteria. If this individual goes to a mental health center, he will be given a "diagnosis" and a prescription for an anxiolytic [a drug used for the treatment of anxiety]. The chances are slim that he will receive any counseling with regards to stress reduction, relationships, or lifestyle. The essential message he receives is that his life and his habits are fine, but that he has a "chemical imbalance" in his brain that is causing him to feel upset and worried, and that the pills will take care of it.

The System Is Broken

In this context, it is important to remember that the vast majority of mental health diagnosing is based on the uncorroborated self-reports of the patient. If you tell a psychiatrist that you are very tense and anxious and that you can't sleep, can't focus on your work, and are irritable with your family—and if you make it sound convincing—you will be given a diagnosis of Generalized Anxiety Disorder and a prescription for an anxiety-reducing drug.

The APA and the pharmaceutical companies have jointly developed this spurious system in which *all* human problems, including normal reactions to stress, are declared mental illnesses which need to be "treated" with drugs. These tactics are focused on people of all ages and all walks of life. Notice in the criteria for generalized anxiety disorder cited above, how much easier it is to assign this diagnosis to a child (one item instead of three).

Anxiety Disorders Are Underdiagnosed and Undertreated

Raymond W. Lam

Raymond W. Lam teaches in the Department of Psychiatry, Faculty of Medicine, University of British Columbia, where he is a professor of psychiatry and head of the Division of Clinical Neuroscience. He is also medical director of the Mood Disorders Centre at UBC Hospital. In this journal article Lam argues that anxiety disorders are highly prevalent in society, yet very often mis- or underdiagnosed and poorly treated. Part of the difficulty lies in the high percentage of patients suffering from other disorders, particularly depression. Lam encourages patients to become active players in their treatment, and points to a wide range of therapies and antianxiety medications that have helped patients improve their clinical outcomes.

Anxiety disorders are highly prevalent in the general population and are the most common of psychiatric conditions. The United States National Comorbidity Survey estimated the cumulative 1-year prevalence rate to be 17% for anxiety disorders, with lifetime prevalence at 25%. Anxiety disorders are associated with considerable morbidity [the prevalence of a particular disease] and disability, and symptoms can vary from mild and transient—without associated impairment—to severe and persistent symptoms that impair function and reduce quality of life.

However, despite their high prevalence and associated impairment, anxiety disorders are frequently unrecognized. Anxiety disorders can have a long duration and recur frequently, and therefore require long-term maintenance treatment. Although there are many effective pharmacological and psychotherapeutic treatments, many patients are under-treated. This paper reviews the treatment challenges in the management of anxiety disorders, the benefits and impact of clinical guidelines, and newer approaches using chronic disease management to optimize treatment.

Challenges in the Management of Anxiety Disorders

The term "anxiety disorder" encompasses a number of different disorders. These disorders can be complicated by the presentation of the many different clinical features of anxiety, leading to difficulties in recognition and diagnosis.

The majority of patients who suffer from anxiety disorders do not access treatment for these problems. A community survey of a major Canadian city revealed that 30% of adults with major depressive disorder (MDD), but only 11% of those with an anxiety disorder, sought help for some form of treatment. Teenagers and young adults were found to be the least likely age group to seek

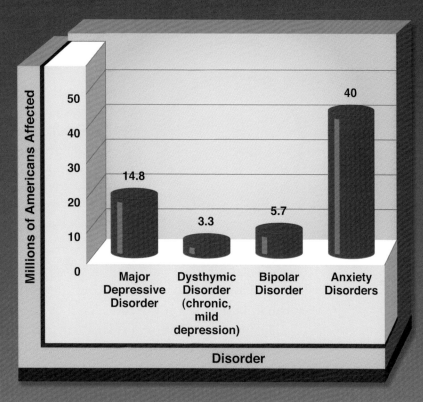

Number of Americans Affected by Mood Disorders and Anxiety Disorders in a Given Year

Millions of Americans Affected

50
40
30
20
10
0

14.8 — Major Depressive Disorder

3.3 — Dysthymic Disorder (chronic, mild depression)

5.7 — Bipolar Disorder

40 — Anxiety Disorders

Disorder

Taken from: National Institute of Mental Health.

mental health resources, despite having a higher likelihood of suffering from these conditions.

Failure to seek treatment is particularly common in patients suffering from social anxiety disorder (SAD), a chronic disorder with an early onset and a low rate of spontaneous recovery (remission of at least 6 months). For example, in a study of 98 patients with SAD (using *DSM-III* [*Diagnostic and Statistical Manual*] criteria) in a North Carolina community, only 32 reported seeing their doctor for psychiatric problems and just three patients admitted to seeking help for their disorder.

A key variable when deciding whether to seek help is the perception of need for treatment. This was shown to be the case in a study of a sample of 1792 patients who were diagnosed with a mood, anxiety, or substance disorder. Only 32% perceived a need for professional help and a minority (19%) actually sought help over a 12-month period. Patients with anxiety disorders alone were about three times less likely to seek help than patients with co-morbid [co-occurring] mood and anxiety disorders. A combination of factors, including psychopathology, various sociodemographic and attitudinal factors appeared to contribute to the reduced perception of need in this patient sample.

Undertreatment

Even when recognized, treatment for anxiety disorders may be less than optimal. This has been demonstrated in a thorough large-scale study conducted by the World Health Organization (WHO) on psychological disorders in primary care. The WHO study screened over 25,000 adults at 15 sites in 14 countries, and over 5000 were further assessed with detailed psychiatric interviews. A quarter had a recognizable mental disorder, the most common being a depressive disorder (11.7%) or an anxiety disorder (10.5%), with 4.6% having both. Only half of the cases of mental disorder were recognized by the primary care physician, and among those, only half were offered treatment. Furthermore, poor patient compliance with medication and inadequate provision of psychotherapy may also occur. In a survey of over 3000 residents in the United States only 14.3% of those with a psychiatric disorder within the past 12 months obtained treatment consistent with evidence-based care recommendations.

FAST FACT

According to the National Institute of Mental Health, most people with one anxiety disorder also have another anxiety disorder.

More than One Disorder

A particular challenge in the management of anxiety disorders is frequent comorbidity; patients often have several coexisting anxiety disorders with overlapping symptoms. In addition, anxiety disorders frequently present with other psychiatric disorders, especially MDD. More than 50% of patients who visit their primary care physician for psychiatric symptoms experience comorbid depression and anxiety, and comorbid conditions are especially common in the elderly. Results from the Zurich epidemiological study found that 48–61% of patients with sporadic panic or panic disorder also suffered from depression within the same year. The prevalence of comorbid generalized anxiety disorder (GAD) and depression, the most common combination, has been reported in as many as 60–90% of patients with GAD in community populations.

Patients who have depression and anxiety comorbidity have higher severity of illness, more chronicity, and significantly greater impairment in work functioning, psychosocial functioning, and quality of life than patients with single diagnoses. Comorbidity also contributes disproportionately to high medical utilization in primary care. For example, the results of the US National Comorbidity Survey demonstrated that anxiety disorder comorbidity was associated with a 2.5-fold increased likelihood of hospitalization. In addition, the longer duration of episodes and higher risk of recurrence associated with comorbidity often requires long-term treatment.

Treatment Guidelines

The good news is that a number of treatments, both pharmacological and psychological, have been found to be effective in treating anxiety disorders. However, it is difficult for busy clinicians to keep up with the many new studies of treatments for complex medical conditions like anxiety disorders. Clinical guidelines can be extremely helpful in summarizing the available evidence base and providing clear recommendations to help clinicians and patients decide on an appropriate course of treatment. Guidelines may also suggest diagnostic schemes to help clinicians explore and identify the type of anxiety disorder and possible comorbidity. For these reasons, guidelines and educational strategies to implement them are increasingly advocated to improve the management of depression and anxiety, especially in primary care.

Unfortunately, despite the effort and resources used in developing and disseminating clinical guidelines, it is unclear whether they have any significant impact on clinical practice. A systematic review of educational and organizational interventions to improve the management of depression in primary care, involving a total of 36 studies, found that simple guidelines implementation and educational strategies were generally ineffective in improving patient outcomes. Other strategies beyond guidelines must be considered to help patients recognize the need for treatment and the importance of treatment adherence, and to help physicians to prepare and engage the patient in the treatment process.

Chronic Disease Management

Anxiety and depression are usually prolonged and recurrent conditions that are rarely "cured" completely and thus may be considered to be chronic. A recent trend in medical care is the development of a proactive approach to chronic disease management (CDM) to improve health outcomes. CDM approaches begin with evidence-based guidelines, but go beyond guidelines to encourage self-management, regular monitoring of outcomes, collaborative care with other health practitioners, and timely access to specialized care. In contrast to guidelines alone, the CDM model has been shown in recent systematic reviews to provide added clinical benefit.

For example, Canadian CDM guidelines for the treatment of MDD in primary care include practical recommendations based on level of evidence, the use of tools such as rating scales and patient education handouts, and a tracking system to register and monitor patients during acute and maintenance phases of treatment. The use of "measurement-based care" has received increasing attention for the treatment of both depression and anxiety, and compilations of rating scales for clinical use in these conditions are now available.

Medications

CDM strategies include simplifying treatments whenever possible. Clinical guidelines give recommendations for many pharmacological agents for the treatment of anxiety disorders. However, practical recommendations for simplifying medication management of anxiety disorders include using broad-spectrum agents and planning for long-term maintenance treatment. Given the comorbidity seen with anxiety disorders, broad-spectrum medications (i.e. those efficacious for several anxiety disorders) should be first considered because not all medications in each class have proven efficacy across the spectrum of anxiety disorders. Since longer-term maintenance treatment for anxiety disorders should be the rule rather than the exception, tolerability is also an important factor to consider when prescribing pharmacological treatment. . . .

Self-Management and Psychotherapy

Most clinical guidelines recommend cognitive behavioral therapy (CBT) as a first-line treatment for many anxiety disorders. CBT in combination with medication is also recommended for refractory symptoms, comorbid conditions, persistent cognitive symptoms, dysfunctional behavioral patterns and anxiety sensitivity. Unfortunately, CBT and other evidence-based psychotherapies are still not widely available to most patients with anxiety

A woman undergoes exposure-based therapy to help overcome her fear of spiders (arachnophobia). (Lea Paterson/Photo Researchers, Inc.)

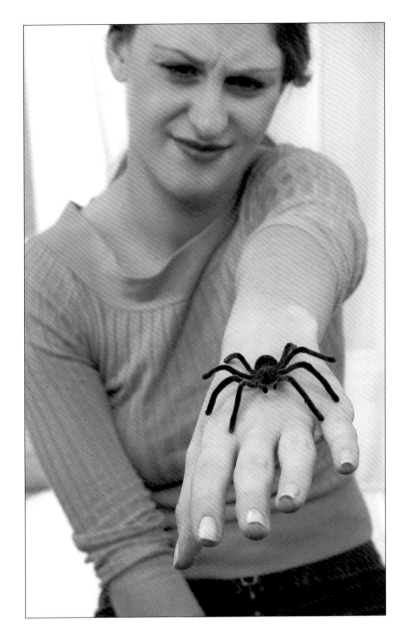

disorders, despite the growing evidence to support their use. The inadequacy of access to psychotherapy may be due to a lack of qualified therapists, physician barriers to recommend evidence-based psychotherapies, and/or lack of funding for non-pharmacological treatments.

Computer-based CBT and self-management programs are novel approaches to delivering psychological treatments. A systematic review of self-help Internet interventions for the treatment of anxiety found
that results were comparable with face-to-face therapy.
One such computer-aided program, FearFighter, has
been recommended for panic disorder in guidelines
from the National Institute for Clinical Excellence in
the United Kingdom. In future, novel approaches such
as these may help to address the shortage of therapists,
thereby improving patient access to evidence-based
psychotherapies.

Anxiety Disorders Need Treatment

Anxiety disorders are highly prevalent, chronic disorders that are frequently under-recognized, misdiagnosed or suboptimally treated. Although clinical
guidelines exist to improve the management of anxiety, guidelines alone are often not effective in improving patient outcomes. Chronic disease management, in conjunction with good clinical guidelines,
can improve these outcomes by focusing on patient
self-management and introducing the use of systems
that help encourage people to obtain the care that they
need. Broad-spectrum antidepressants with proven efficacy in the treatment of both anxiety and depression
are first-line agents for anxiety disorders, and selec-
tion of medication should consider both efficacy and
long-term tolerability. Although combination therapy
involving medication and CBT has been shown to be
useful, the availability of psychotherapy is currently
limited. Computer-based programs delivered via the
Internet may represent a novel method to increase access to evidence-based psychological treatment. Together, these strategies should help improve clinical
outcomes in patients with anxiety disorders.

Social Anxiety Disorder Is Not Just Shyness

Martin A. Katzman

In this article from the *Journal of Family Practice* Martin A. Katzman explains that social anxiety disorder is a surprisingly prevalent and debilitating condition that is more severe than simple shyness. If not diagnosed and treated, patients suffering from this disorder have a higher tendency to develop substance abuse problems and depression. Katzman clarifies the symptoms, screening tools, therapies, and drug options for social anxiety disorder patients and emphasizes that early diagnosis is crucial to achieving positive outcomes.

Katzman is the clinical director at the START (Stress, Trauma, Anxiety Rehabilitation and Treatment) Clinic for Mood and Anxiety Disorders as well as a staff psychiatrist at the Centre for Addiction and Mental Health–Clarke Division. Both facilities are located in Toronto, Canada. His research studies examine the psychobiological and cognitive processes in mood and anxiety disorders.

SOURCE: Martin A. Katzman, "Beyond Shy: When to Suspect Social Anxiety Disorder," *Journal of Family Practice*, vol. 56, May 2007, pp. 369–74. Copyright © 2007 Dowden Health Media, Inc. Reproduced by permission.

Janice L, 41, comes into her physician's office complaining that she's "feeling anxious all the time" at her job at a local bank. She tells him that she's been treated for depression in the past, though she's not currently taking any antidepressants. As her physician takes a more thorough history, he notices that her alcohol consumption seems a bit excessive. Her demeanor, which he had previously chalked up to as "shyness," comes into focus. He begins to suspect that his patient is more than just "quiet and unassuming" and may, in fact, be suffering from social anxiety disorder.

To confirm his suspicions, he excuses himself to retrieve an article he'd saved on the topic—one that identifies a quick screening tool for social anxiety disorder. He then asks his patient to rate the following statements on a scale of 0 to 4, with 0 being "not at all" and 4 being "extremely present":

- Fear of embarrassment causes me to avoid doing things or speaking to people.
- I avoid activities in which I am the center of attention.
- Being embarrassed or looking stupid are among my worst fears.

His suspicions are confirmed when she scores a 10—well above the 6 that is highly suggestive of social anxiety disorder.

A Common Disorder

Social anxiety, also known as social phobia, is the most common anxiety disorder, and is the third most common psychiatric disorder after depression and alcohol dependence. The Epidemiological Catchment Area Study [by the National Institute of Mental Health] revealed that 2% to 4% of the sample suffered from social anxiety with a lifetime prevalence of 2.8%. Other studies have found that as many at 10% of the sample suffer from social anxiety when a more appropriate diagnostic

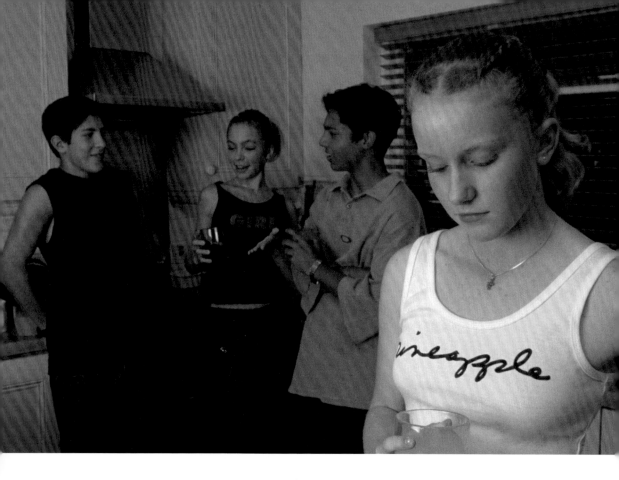

Social anxiety disorder is characterized by a fear of social interactions and of negative evaluations by others. (© Bubbles Photolibrary/Alamy)

interview is used. Similarly, [a study by R.C. Kessler and Associates] investigating the prevalence of *DSM-IV* [*Diagnostic and Statistical Manual*] disorders and concluded that 6.8% of the entire sample suffered from social anxiety disorder.

Social anxiety disorder is characterized as a persistent and debilitating fear of social interaction where patients fear negative evaluations by others. As a result, these patients may have trouble building and maintaining social relationships, which can result in a particularly isolated and depressed lifestyle.

Subtypes

There are 2 subtypes of social anxiety disorder:

- Generalized social anxiety is generally more severe and more generalized and, therefore, more disabling to patients. The majority of patients seen by the medical community tend to exhibit this subtype of the disorder.

• Nongeneralized anxiety (also known as specific or discrete social phobia) is the less common and usually includes a fear associated with 1 or a few specific situations.

Although nongeneralized anxiety may be less likely to cause severe impairment in the patient's life, it still may lead to significant underachievement in school or work. Still, patients with public speaking–only social anxiety are more likely to recover spontaneously, while patients with generalized social anxiety rarely recover spontaneously from the disorder.

The 2 subtypes also differ in their origin. Generalized social anxiety—the focus of this article—is significantly more prevalent among relatives who also suffer from the disorder, while patients with nongeneralized social anxiety disorder do not necessarily have relatives with the condition.

Not Just Shyness

Social anxiety is a lifelong disorder that may begin as early as childhood, but is often described as beginning at age 13. At this age, though, the social anxiety is often mistaken for extreme shyness and therefore goes untreated.

The difference between social anxiety disorder and shyness in children is that social anxiety debilitates the child's ability to grow and develop socially in an appropriate manner. While children with—and without— social anxiety disorder may be uncomfortable around unfamiliar adults, children with this disorder will also be uncomfortable in a peer setting with unfamiliar kids their own age. Children with social anxiety may express their discomfort through crying, tantrums, or freezing from the social situation. In order for the child to meet full criteria for social anxiety, the duration of the symptoms must span at least 6 months.

Overlooking shyness in such a young patient is particularly problematic as the avoidance that characterizes the social anxiety disorder can result in a lost opportunity to acquire social skills that are needed to ease the transition from adolescence to adulthood. This relative loss of social skills often facilitates the development of social dysfunction that is characteristic of this illness. As time goes by, sufferers eventually become accustomed to their fears and create a way of life that accommodates them.

Life Complications

Social anxiety can interrupt education or job success, cause financial dependence, and impair relationships. Sufferers tend to miss out on important social events and activities in their lives, and they begin to accumulate comorbidities [co-occurring conditions] such as depression and substance abuse. In fact, while many cases of social anxiety are overlooked as shyness, others are misdiagnosed as depression.

Complicating matters further is the issue of substance abuse. The Epidemiological Catchment Area Study found that alcohol abuse was reported in 17% of social anxiety cases and drug abuse was reported in 13%. In the study conducted by Kessler et al, results indicated that 8.8% of individuals suffering from a substance abuse problem also suffered from comorbid social anxiety.

The substance abuse evolves slowly, and tends to arise as an inappropriate coping mechanism because so many cases of social anxiety go untreated.

Symptoms

The primary indicator of social anxiety is intense fear of social situations. A patient suffering from social anxiety fears that he or she will act in a way that will be humiliating when confronted with unfamiliar situations or people or by the possibility of being scrutinized by others. While many people with social anxiety realize that their fears are excessive or unreasonable, they are unable to overcome them.

There are also a number of physical, cognitive, and behavioral symptoms that are associated with social anxiety. The physical symptoms may include rapid heart rate, trembling, shortness of breath, sweating, and abdominal pain. The cognitive symptoms include maladaptive thoughts and beliefs about social situations (ie, irrational thought processes), that increase the anxiety when in the situation. Finally, behavioral symptoms include phobic avoidance of the feared situation.

> **FAST FACT**
>
> The Anxiety Disorders Association of America states that 15 million Americans suffer from social anxiety disorder. It is equally common among men and women.

Screening Devices

There are many screening devices that [a physician] can use to identify patients with social anxiety disorder or to assess the severity of symptoms. Some examples include the Liebowitz Social Phobia Scale, the Social Phobia Inventory (SPIN), Fear of Negative Evaluation Scale, and the Social Avoidance and Distress Scale. These tools, however, can be a bit time consuming.

A more handy—though admittedly less comprehensive—screening device is the "mini SPIN." . . . In a study of 7165 managed care patients, 89% of the cases meeting criteria for social anxiety disorder were detected (with a score of 6 or better) using this screening method.

To review, [a doctor needs] to ask patients to rate the following statements on a scale of 0 "not at all" to 4 "extremely present":

  1. Fear of embarrassment causes me to avoid doing things or speaking to people.

2. I avoid activities in which I am the center of attention.

3. Being embarrassed or looking stupid are among my worst fears.

A score of 6 or higher should prompt [the physician] to further evaluate the patient using one of the screening devices listed earlier.

Social Anxiety Disorder Treatments

Although social anxiety most commonly spans a lifetime, studies indicate that treatment—typically cognitive behavioral therapy (CBT) with drug therapy—can help sufferers deal with their fears and function more efficiently in their everyday lives. The best effects in treating

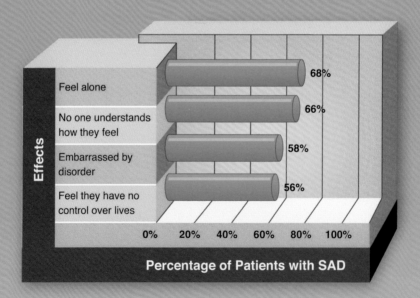

Effects of Social Anxiety Disorders (SAD) on Patients

Taken from: Anxiety Disorders Association of America.

social anxiety, therefore, are in combining the different treatment strategies.

Cognitive Behavioral Therapy

[Psychology researcher Richard] Heimberg and colleagues found that 75% of social anxiety patients who participated in a cognitive behavioral therapy group experienced improved function and saw a reduction in symptoms of social anxiety. Successful CBT seems to not only alleviate symptomatic distress, but improve the patients' perceptions of their general quality of life. Including behavioral components such as reinforcement or conditioning in CBT appears to be effective in helping sufferers minimize their symptoms. In addition, cognitive restructuring (ie, changing a patient's thought process) has also been shown to be a helpful treatment.

Some of the basic elements of CBT include anxiety management skills (ie, breathing and relaxation techniques), social skills training (ie, maintaining conversation with the patient while monitoring the patient's eye contact), and gradual exposure to the feared situation (ie, exposure to social situations).

Drug Therapy

Studies have also demonstrated the effectiveness of a variety of medications (including Venlafaxine XR [Effexor XR], Paroxetine [Paxil], Paroxetine CR [Paxil CR], Sertraline [Zoloft], and Fluvoxamine [Luvox]) in managing social anxiety disorder. If [a doctor is] caring for a patient with social anxiety disorder, [he or she will] want to start him on a selective serotonin reuptake inhibitor (SSRI) or serotonin-norepinephrine reuptake inhibitor (SNRI).

If this doesn't achieve the desired results, the next step is a monoamine oxidase inhibitor, such as phenelzine (Nardil), or a reverse inhibitor of monoamine oxidase A, such as moclobemide. Additionally, some benzodiazepines and anticonvulsants (clonazepam [Klonopin] and pregabalin [Lyrica]) may also be effective if the other options do not achieve the desired results. . . .

When putting [a] patient on any of these medications, patient teaching will be important. [A physician needs] to advise the patient that common antidepressant side effects include, but are not limited to, nausea, diarrhea, sexual dysfunction (ie, delayed orgasm), and headaches. These effects, however, typically disappear by the second week of intake. If the patient is taking a benzodiazepine, [he or she needs to be warned] about the risk of psychomotor or cognitive impairment.

If the patient has a comorbid substance abuse problem, [the physician] and the patient will also need to adjust expectations somewhat. That's because patients with a substance abuse problem are likely to have a poorer response to some of these medications than patients without a substance abuse problem.

Though the time it takes to manage the condition is variable, patients with social anxiety disorder can improve their situation and go on to live more fulfilling and happy lives. The trick, really, is spotting the disorder early, rather than assuming [a] patient is simply the "quiet type."

Social Anxiety Disorder and Shyness Are Similar

Roger Dobson

In this British newspaper article from the *Times* (London), Roger Dobson questions the legitimacy of turning shyness into a medical disorder. Instead of teaching people to be comfortable with their natural, reserved personalities, society seems to be telling them that they have an unhealthy state of mind requiring therapies and drugs as treatment. This is particularly worrisome to some researchers seeing a rise in the number of shy people due to a technological revolution that has isolated individuals and to the smaller size of modern families. Dobson concludes his article by emphasizing the importance of being yourself in a world that too often forces people to conform to a single, more outgoing standard.

Dobson is a British journalist who has written articles for the *Independent*, *MailOnline*, the *Daily Telegraph*, the *Times*, the *Sunday Times*, and the *Sunday Telegraph*.

Goodbye shyness, hello avoidant-personality disorder. Shyness, once an accepted and even admired trait, has been hijacked and given the status of a syndrome. Some experts believe that half the population now "suffer" from it. But is it natural or a medical affliction?

"Social phobia" was recognised as a diagnosis in 1980 and, since then, it has been joined in the textbooks by social-anxiety disorder and avoidant-personality disorder. For those deemed to be afflicted there is counselling available as well as self-help books, hypnotherapy and psychotherapy. And for severe cases, there are drugs—mainly antidepressants, but also beta-blockers and botulinum toxin (for the excess sweating caused by shyness). There are even half a dozen shyness clinics around the country.

But not everyone agrees that shyness is a medical affliction. A conference next week [April 2006] of academics and health professionals in Newcastle, New South Wales, will debate the rise of "disease-mongering". Some delegates will argue that defining natural conditions as diseases is merely a way for pharmaceutical companies to make money from the well. Health practitioners on the fringe of mainstream medicine also profit from this trend.

Making Shyness into a Disorder

New research published by the University of Sussex is adding fuel to the debate.

It suggests that we have gone too far with making shyness into a disorder. The researchers say it's more about society being uneasy with those who don't conform to the assertive, gregarious standards of the 21st century, than actually helping people. "Shyness has become an unhealthy state of mind for individuals living in contemporary Western societies," says Dr Susie Scott, a sociologist at Sussex University who led the research. "The increasing medicalisation of shyness suggests that bashful modesty and reserve are no longer

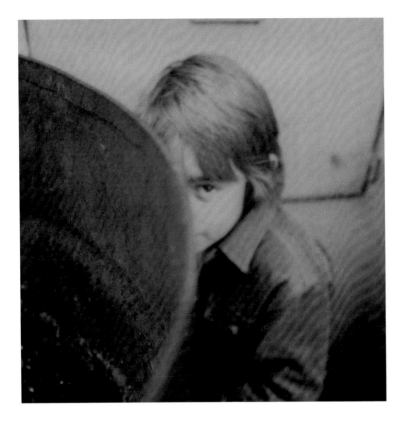

New research at the University of Sussex casts doubt on whether shyness is a social disorder. (© PhotoAlto/Alamy)

so acceptable and that to succeed we must be vocal, assertive and capable of gregariously participating in social life. As shyness becomes less socially acceptable, the shyest people are finding that their identities are being recast in biomedical terms and subjected to psychiatric treatment."

Shy people are increasingly directed towards talking therapies, says Dr Scott, in which they are taught that their tendency towards quietness, passivity and withdrawal in social situations will not do and that it must be unlearnt.

"By producing a steady flow of re-socialised, conformist 'gingerbread men', therapeutic regimes perpetuate the idea that non-shyness is both a normal and a desirable state to be in and that shy people have an obligation to change," says a report of the research, which will be appearing shortly in the journal *Sociology of Health and Illness.*

Accepting Shyness

Why shyness is no longer acceptable is debatable. Dr Bernado Carducci, the head of the Shyness Research Institute, at the University of Indiana, says that the speed of modern life doesn't allow shy people the time they need to warm up.

But many shy people are resisting the medicalisation and what American researchers call "cosmetic psychopharmacology", the use of drugs to change natural traits.

There are now a number of internet sites claiming that shyness is a positive, life-affirming experience. A website for AOL members asserts that shyness is who you are. One contributor says: "I have noticed that there are programmes to treat shyness as if it were a disease. Shyness is not a disease. Shy people are probably the most kind-hearted people there are. Be thankful for it."

Causes Are Not Clear

It's still not clear what causes shyness. The latest thinking suggests that it is an over-the-top response to fear of people thinking negatively about you. Research at Stanford University suggests that although there may be a genetic predisposition to shyness in some people, most shyness is triggered by early life experiences, such as insecurity, frequent criticism, a dominant sibling, family conflict and stress at school.

The first signs that shyness was no longer being seen as just a personality trait came three decades ago when Philip Zimbardo and Lynne Henderson, at Stanford University, found that 40 per cent of those who took part in a survey described themselves as chronically shy, with a further 15 per cent shy in some situations.

They have now updated the prevalence rate to 50 per cent. "We may want to take note of increasing levels of shyness as a warning of a public health danger that appears to be heading toward epidemic proportions," they said last year [2005].

Symptoms of Shyness

Behavioral

Inhibition and passivity
Gaze aversion
Avoidance of feared situations
Low speaking voice
Little body movement or expression or excessive nodding or smiling
Speech dysfluencies
Nervous behaviors, such as touching one's hair or face

Physiological

Accelerated heart rate
Dry mouth
Trembling or shaking
Sweating
Feeling faint or dizzy, butterflies in stomach or nausea
Experiencing the situation or oneself as unreal or removed
Fear of losing control, going crazy, or having a heart attack

Cognitive

Negative thoughts about the self, the situation, and others
Fear of negative evaluation and looking foolish to others
Worry and rumination, perfectionism
Self-blaming attributions, particularly after social interaction
Negative beliefs about the self (weak) and others (powerful), often out of awareness
Negative biases in the self-concept, e.g., "I am socially inadequate, unlovable, unattractive."
A belief that there is a "correct" protocol that the shy person must guess, rather than mutual definitions of social situations

Affective

Embarrassment and painful self-consciousness
Shame
Low self-esteem
Dejection and sadness
Loneliness
Depression
Anxiety

Confusing Personality with a Disorder

That growing sense of alarm about shyness has coincided with the increasing availability of drugs, the arrival of shyness clinics, a proliferation of talking therapy, and the reported discovery of culprit genes. All of which means that it has been increasingly regarded as a modifiable disease.

That's certainly the approach at the London Shyness Centre, which uses neurolinguistic programming, psychotherapy and hypnotherapy to help shy people. A brochure for patients says: "Confident people with high self-esteem are able to pursue their dreams and goals, they feel worthy of their achievements. This can be you. Be everything you ever dreamt of being."

But the key question in the great shyness debate is when—if ever—does a personality trait become a medical disorder? With most personality traits there is a case for treating people whose extreme behaviour is problematic to themselves and others. But the creeping medicalisation of a whole personality trait in its own right is another matter. Perhaps it is not surprising that the move towards increased medicalisation comes at a time when the proportion of the population estimated to be shy is tipped to rise. Home working, computers and internet based activities have all led to less socialising and less practice for social skills.

"Shyness has got worse because of two revolutions," says Dr Elizabeth Morris, the principal of the School of Emotional Literacy, a consultancy in Gloucestershire [England], that advises schools on children's emotional issues. "There has been a technological revolution, which means that children are interacting with screens rather than people, so neglecting to use social skills.

"The second revolution has occurred in families, which are now much smaller, and where it is not very

FAST FACT

Abraham Lincoln, Thomas Edison, and Albert Einstein were all shy at one time in their lives.

common for children to sit and eat meals at a table with parents or carers. It happens once a week on average now, so the everyday possibilities for natural social intercourse are much less." In that case, could shyness become not a deviancy but the norm? As one contributor to an online shyness noticeboard suggests, shouldn't it be the group that is becoming the minority—the socially skilled, assertive, extroverts—who are offered pills and psychotherapy to make them less forthcoming?

Be Yourself

It seems unlikely. But the shy can at least find some solace from the author Jerome K. Jerome, a self-confessed shy man, who advised against trying to find a cure for the affliction. He wrote: "Your attempt to put on any other disposition than your own will infallibly result in your becoming ridiculously gushing and offensively familiar. Be your own natural self, and then you will only be thought to be surly and stupid."

Post-Traumatic Stress Disorder Is Underdiagnosed

Michael de Yoanna and Mark Benjamin

In this article for the online magazine *Salon*, Michael de Yoanna and Mark Benjamin investigate the U.S. military's efforts to stop its medical staff from diagnosing post-traumatic stress disorder (PTSD) among its troops. Focusing on one anonymous sergeant's struggle to have his symptoms recognized and treated, the authors build their case to encompass a larger scandal, from the physicians offering alternative and weaker diagnoses to the authorities ordering them to do so. Because of the high cost in offering PTSD sufferers disability payments for their injuries, the authors believe that there is a concerted attempt to avoid the financial drain on the military at the expense of those soldiers traumatized in battle.

A journalist whose news investigations and features have won twelve professional awards, De Yoanna is currently the chief facilitator/moderator for MileHive.com. Benjamin is a national correspondent with *Salon* and has written extensively on the subject of the war wounded.

SOURCE: Michael de Yoanna and Mark Benjamin, "I Am Under a Lot of Pressure to Not Diagnose PTSD," *Salon*, April 8, 2009. This article first appeared in Salon.com, at www.salon.com. An online version remains in the Salon archives. Reprinted with permission.

"Sgt. X" is built like the Bradley Fighting Vehicle he rode in while in Iraq. He's as bulky, brawny and seemingly impervious as a tank.

In an interview in the high-rise offices of his Denver attorneys, however, symptoms of the damaged brain inside that tough exterior begin to appear. Sgt. X's eyes go suddenly blank, shifting to refocus oddly on a wall. He pauses mid-sentence, struggling for simple words. His hands occasionally tremble and spasm.

For more than a year he's been seeking treatment at Fort Carson for a brain injury and post-traumatic stress disorder [PTSD], the signature injuries of the Iraq war. Sgt. X is also suffering through the Army's confusing disability payment system, handled by something called a medical evaluation board. The process of negotiating the system has been made harder by his war-damaged memory. Sgt. X's wife has to go with him to doctor's appointments so he'll remember what the doctor tells him.

The Military's Push Against PTSD

But what Sgt. X wants to tell a reporter about is one doctor's appointment at Fort Carson that his wife did not witness. When she couldn't accompany him to an appointment with psychologist Douglas McNinch last June [2008], Sgt. X tucked a recording device into his pocket and set it on voice-activation so it would capture what the doctor said. Sgt. X had no idea that the little machine in his pocket was about to capture recorded evidence of something wounded soldiers and their advocates have long suspected—that the military does not want Iraq veterans to be diagnosed with PTSD, a condition that obligates the military to provide expensive, intensive long-term care, including the possibility of lifetime disability payments. And . . . after the Army became aware of the tape, the Senate Armed Services Committee declined to investigate its implications, despite prodding

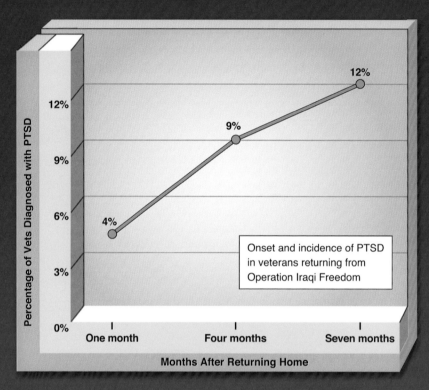

Post-Traumatic Stress Disorder (PTSD) in the Iraq War

Percentage of Vets Diagnosed with PTSD

12%

9%

6%

3%

0%

12%

9%

4%

One month   Four months   Seven months

Months After Returning Home

Onset and incidence of PTSD in veterans returning from Operation Iraqi Freedom

Taken from: http://ptsdcombat.blogspot.com/2007/03/war-list-oefoif-statistics.html.

from a senator who is not on the committee. The Army then conducted its own internal investigation—and cleared itself of any wrongdoing.

When Sgt. X went to see McNinch with a tape recorder, he was concerned that something was amiss with his diagnosis. He wanted to find out why the psychologist had told the medical evaluation board that handles disability payments that Sgt. X did not, in fact, have PTSD, but instead an "anxiety disorder," which could substantially lower the amount of benefits he would receive if the Army discharged him for a disability. The recorder in Sgt. X's pocket captured McNinch in a moment of candor.

"OK," McNinch told Sgt. X. "I will tell you something confidentially that I would have to deny if it were ever public. Not only myself, but all the clinicians up here are being pressured to not diagnose PTSD and diagnose anxiety disorder NOS [not otherwise specified] [instead]." McNinch told him that Army medical boards were "kick[ing] back" his diagnoses of PTSD, saying soldiers had not seen enough trauma to have "serious PTSD issues."

"Unfortunately," McNinch told Sgt. X, "yours has not been the only case. . . . I and other [doctors] are under a lot of pressure to not diagnose PTSD. It's not fair. I think it's a horrible way to treat soldiers, but unfortunately, you know, now the V.A. [Department of Veteran Affairs] is jumping on board, saying, 'Well, these people don't have PTSD,' and stuff like that."

Pressured Not to Diagnose

Contacted recently by *Salon*, McNinch seemed surprised that reporters had obtained the tape, but answered questions about the statements captured by the recording. McNinch told *Salon* that the pressure to misdiagnose came from the former head of Fort Carson's Department of Behavioral Health. That colonel, an Army psychiatrist, is now at Fort Lewis in Washington State. "This was pressure that the commander of my Department of Behavioral Health put on me at that time," he said. Since McNinch is a civilian employed by the Army, the colonel could not *order* him to give a specific, lesser diagnosis to soldiers. Instead, McNinch said, the colonel would "refuse to concur with me, or argue with me, or berate me" when McNinch diagnosed soldiers with PTSD. "It is just very difficult being a civilian in a military setting."

McNinch added that he also received pressure not to properly diagnose traumatic brain injury, Sgt. X's other medical problem. "When I got there I was told I was overdiagnosing brain injuries and now everybody is finding out that, yes, there are brain injuries," he recalled. McNinch said he argued, "'What are we going to do about treatment?' And they said, 'Oh, we are just counting people. We don't plan on treating them.'" McNinch replied, "'You are bringing a generation of brain-damaged individuals back here. You have got to get a game plan together for this public health crisis.'"

When McNinch learned he would be quoted in a *Salon* article, he cut off further questions. He also said he would deny the interview took place. *Salon*, however, had recorded the conversation.

On the tape and in his interview with *Salon*, McNinch seemed to admit what countless soldiers not just at Fort Carson but across the Army have long suspected: At least in some cases, the Army tries to avoid diagnoses of PTSD. But McNinch did not directly address why the Army discourages these diagnoses, in either the interview with *Salon* or the tape-recorded encounter with Sgt. X.

Financial Costs of Diagnosing

The answer probably has to do with money. David Rudd, the chairman of Texas Tech's department of psychology and a former Army psychologist, explained that every dollar the Army spends on a soldier's benefits is a dollar lost for bullets, bombs or the soldier's incoming replacement. "Each diagnosis is an acknowledgment that psychiatric casualties are a huge price tag of this war," said Rudd. "It is easiest to dismiss these casualties because you can't see the wounds. If they change the diagnosis they can dismiss you at a substantially decreased rate."

A recently retired Army psychiatrist who still works for the government, speaking on the condition of anonymity for fear of retribution, said commanders at another Army hospital instructed him to misdiagnose soldiers suffering from war-related PTSD, recommending instead that he diagnose them with other disorders that would reduce their benefits. The psychiatrist said he

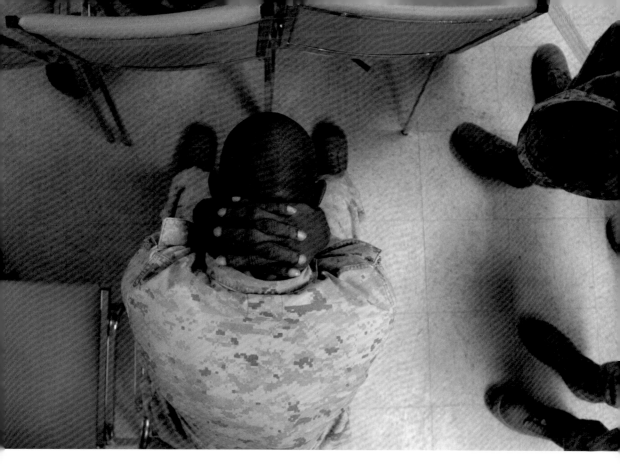

would be willing to say more publicly about the cases and provide specific names, but only if President [Barack] Obama would protect him from retaliation.

A soldier awaits psychological testing for post-traumatic stress disorder. Critics say the army is systematically trying to avoid paying for treatment of the disorder by minimizing its impact on soldiers. (AP Images)

A Soldier's Reluctance to Speak

Salon has dubbed the soldier in this article Sgt. X because he asked not to be identified for fear that it might affect the medical evaluation process meant to gauge his level of disability. He was highly reluctant to speak, but agreed to do so after learning *Salon* obtained the recording and other information about it from a medical worker at Fort Carson and a congressional aide.

The sergeant spoke with *Salon* in the presence of his Hogan & Hartson attorneys who are helping him to secure a proper disability discharge from the Army for PTSD and a brain injury, diagnoses now affirmed by independent doctors. Sgt. X never planned to go to the media—he says, if asked, he will not talk further about the recording with news organizations.

Sgt. X probably received his traumatic brain injury when his Bradley Fighting Vehicle buckled in an explosion during his second deployment to Iraq in 2005–06. It was the worst of a handful of nearby blasts he'd survived, and it knocked him unconscious for 30 seconds.

When Sgt. X regained consciousness, he saw that the toes of another soldier had been sheared off. The tank hull had buckled and the inside had filled with smoke. Some of his fellow soldiers were soaked in blood.

Even after that, as a point of pride, the crew insisted on accompanying their disabled tank back to their headquarters. Besides causing his brain injury, the blast had exacerbated an injury to Sgt. X's hip, but he faced the problem with little complaint. He numbed the pain with Motrin. "You don't report problems," he said. "It's a stigma."

When Sgt. X returned from the war to Colorado Springs, though, he had a problem with anger. After he terrified his young son by screaming at him, Sgt. X's wife suggested he seek help.

Nearly breaking into tears while recounting the screaming bout to *Salon*, Sgt. X said he agreed to his wife's request and sought mental care for the first time in his 16-year military career. Sgt. X, like so many others on the post, went to the fourth floor of Evans Hospital in search of mental-health assistance.

A Larger Scandal

There is some evidence that Sgt. X's experience with Mc-Ninch represents part of a broader scandal, as suggested by the former Army psychiatrist who told *Salon* about identical problems at another post. Last year [in 2008], VoteVets.org and Citizens for Responsibility and Ethics in Washington (CREW) released an e-mail from Norma Perez, a psychologist in Texas, to staff at a Department of Veterans Affairs facility there. In addition to the Army, that department also provides veterans with benefits "Given that we are having more and more compensation seeking veterans, I'd like to suggest that you refrain from giving a diagnosis of PTSD straight out," Perez wrote in the e-mail dated March 20, 2008. She suggested the staff "consider a diagnosis of Adjustment Disorder." As opposed to those with PTSD, veterans with adjustment disorder, a temporary condition, typically do not receive disability payments from the government.

Then-Illinois Sen. Barack Obama fired a letter off to the V.A. about that previous controversy, calling the e-mail "outrageous," demanding an investigation. The Senate Veterans' Affairs Committee last June held a hearing on that e-mail, Perez claimed she sent that e-mail "to stress the importance of an accurate diagnosis." End of story.

> **FAST FACT**
>
> The diagnosis of PTSD first appeared in 1980 in the *Diagnostic and Statistical Manual* of the American Psychiatric Association.

VoteVets.org and CREW, the two groups who unearthed the V.A. e-mail, reacted viscerally to this new tape obtained by *Salon*. "This is further evidence our troops are not receiving the mental health treatment they need and deserve," said Melanie Sloan, CREW executive director. "The president and congressional leaders must hold those responsible accountable and make sure the message is sent far and wide that our returning troops are to be diagnosed as their symptoms, not the military's finances, dictate."

"We've heard all kinds of stories from vets who had trouble getting PTSD diagnoses," said VoteVets.org Chairman John Soltz. "It's crucial that we have department-wide investigations at the Departments of Defense and Veterans Affairs to determine if this came from someone high up, and how many troops and veterans were jilted out of a proper diagnosis from the government."

More Examples of Underdiagnosis

Many publications, including *Salon*, and even some government agencies have documented other instances of reluctance to recognize mental wounds caused by war at bases across the country.

- A recent weeklong series in *Salon* showed how apparent resistance to identifying combat stress ends up grinding down the lowest-ranking troops, sometimes with deadly results. Those articles included, for example, the story of Pvt. Adam Lieberman, who suffered with severe symptoms of PTSD. For two years, the Army blamed his problems on a personality disorder, anxiety disorder or alcohol abuse but resisted diagnosing him with PTSD until after his suicide attempt last October [2008].
- The Government Accountability Office, Congress' investigative arm, last October questioned why 2,800 war veterans were labeled with personality disorder diagnoses, another cheap label the Army has been accused of plastering on soldiers instead of PTSD.
- In November 2005 the Department of Veterans Affairs halted a review of 72,000 veterans who receive monthly disability payments for mental trauma from war. The department wanted to make sure the veterans were not faking their symptoms. *Salon* first exposed the review that August. Then Daniel L. Cooper, the V.A.'s undersecretary for benefits, told *Salon* at the time that, "We have a responsibility to preserve the integrity of the rating system and to ensure that hard-earned taxpayer dollars are going to those who deserve and have earned them." The department stopped the process a month after a Vietnam veteran in New Mexico, agitated over the review, shot himself to death in protest.
- In early 2005, *Salon* exposed a pattern of medical officials searching to pin soldiers' problems on childhood trauma instead of combat stress at Walter Reed Army Medical Center.

Post-Traumatic Stress Disorder Is Overdiagnosed

Daniel J. Carlat

Daniel J. Carlat is assistant clinical professor of psychiatry at Tufts University School of Medicine and also maintains a private practice. He is editor in chief of the *Carlat Psychiatry Report*, a monthly newsletter that provides clinically relevant information on psychiatric practice without any funding from the pharmaceutical industry.

In this 2007 article the author argues that while post-traumatic stress disorder (PTSD) is certainly a valid diagnosis to assign to many patients, its diagnostic criteria have become too loosely defined. The diagnosis has therefore been assigned to patients whose symptoms do not reach the severity of those who are truly suffering as the result of directly experiencing a past traumatic event. As a consequence, the ranks of PTSD patients have swelled since Vietnam, as has the government spending on their care. The author advocates for a tighter set of PTSD diagnostic criteria in the future and for more caution to be exercised by physicians in their diagnoses.

SOURCE: Daniel J. Carlat, "PTSD: Is It 'Real'?" *The Carlat Psychiatry Report*, vol. 5, June 2007, pp. 1–2. Copyright © 2007 Clearview Publishing, LLC. All rights reserved. Reproduced by permission.

A recent issue of the *Journal of Anxiety Disorders* (Vol. 21, 2007) focused on the troubling possibility that the PTSD (posttraumatic stress disorder) construct is not nearly as valid as has been assumed. The articles are both fascinating and provocative and are well worth reading.

The Findings

The journal kicks off with a bombshell of a study by [Dr. Alexander Bodkin] and his colleagues at McLean Hospital. The researchers enrolled 103 subjects who had originally been recruited for clinical trials of anti-depressants. As part of the original study protocol, all patients were administered the Structured Clinical Interview for DSM-IV [*Diagnostic and Statistical Manual of Mental Disorders*] Axis I Disorders (SCID). The SCID has a section on PTSD, which instructs raters to first ask patients if they have ever experienced a traumatic event ("criterion A"). If the patient responds positively, you ask about the remaining criteria (B–F) in turn, but if there has not been a trauma, you are to skip the questions and code the patient as not having the diagnosis.

In this fiendishly clever study, however, raters asked about criteria B-F *even if there was no traumatic event*. This is not as easy as it sounds; for example, how does one ask about flashbacks or nightmares in the absence of a traumatic event? To get around this, researchers asked subjects to think about something they had been worrying about, and then referred to this worry when they asked the questions. For example: "Have you had any nightmares about the possibility that you might have to declare bankruptcy," and so on. What were the results? Of the 103 subjects, 54 had experienced a traumatic event, and of these, 42 (78%) of them also met symptomatic criteria for PTSD. Thirty six patients had never experienced trauma, and when these nontraumatized patients were interviewed, fully 28 (also 78%) met all the remaining criteria (B through F) for PTSD.

Diagnostic Criteria for Post-Traumatic Stress Disorder

A. Exposure to a traumatic event

1. Response involves intense fear, helplessness, or horror

B. Traumatic event is persistently reexperienced in at least one of the following ways:

1. Recurrent and intrusive thoughts or images
2. Recurrent distressing dreams
3. Acting or feeling as if the event were recurring
4. Psychological distress upon exposure to reminders of event
5. Physiological reactions upon exposure to reminders of event

C. Avoidance of stimuli associated with the event and numbing of general response, occurring in at least three of the following ways:

1. Efforts to avoid thoughts, feelings, or conversations about the event
2. Efforts to avoid activities, places, or people that remind person of the event
3. Inability to remember an important aspect of the event
4. Significantly diminished interest or participation in activities
5. Feeling of being detached or estranged from others
6. Restricted range of affect
7. Speaks or thinks of not having a future

D. increased arousal not present before traumatic event, presenting in at least two of the following ways:

1. Trouble falling or staying asleep
2. Irritability or outbursts of anger
3. Difficulty concentrating
4. Hypervigilance
5. Exaggerated startle response

E. Symptoms last at least one month

F. Symptoms listed above cause significant impairment in daily life

Taken from: *Diagnostic and Statistical Manual of Mental Disorders (IV)*.

PTSD's Surging Popularity

The implication is that PTSD is not necessarily a "post-traumatic" disorder, but rather a non-specific cluster of symptoms that often occur with or without trauma. In the authors' words: "It would follow, therefore, that in patients manifesting the symptom cluster of PTSD, it may be hazardous to assume that these symptoms were caused by trauma, even if an unequivocal traumatic event occurred."

But if PTSD is so non-specific, why did the diagnosis become so popular? In another article in the same issue, [researchers Paul McHugh and Glenn Treisman] of Johns Hopkins trace the history and genesis of the PTSD concept. Surprisingly, the first formal definition of PTSD did not occur until 1980, with the publication of *DSM-3*. However, army doctors had known for decades that traumatic events often led to a syndrome that included emotional numbness, anxiety, flashbacks, and nightmares. World War I military doctors treated "shell shock" with brief removal from the combat zone and with psychotherapy emphasizing that the reactions were normal responses to combat and would soon dissipate.

The authors trace the ascendancy of "PTSD" to the Vietnam war. In their opinion, the diagnosis of PTSD in Vietnam veterans served several purposes at once. Veterans found a PTSD diagnosis less stigmatizing than alternative diagnoses, such as alcoholism and personality disorders. As an institution, the Veteran's Administration found the diagnosis useful in expanding its own bureaucracy and ensuring continued funding for specialized PTSD treatment units.

After Vietnam

After Vietnam, the ranks of PTSD patients swelled, and in 1983, Congress, alarmed at how much government money was being spent on PTSD treatment, commissioned a special study of its prevalence. The results, released in 1988, showed that almost a million of the 3.14 million

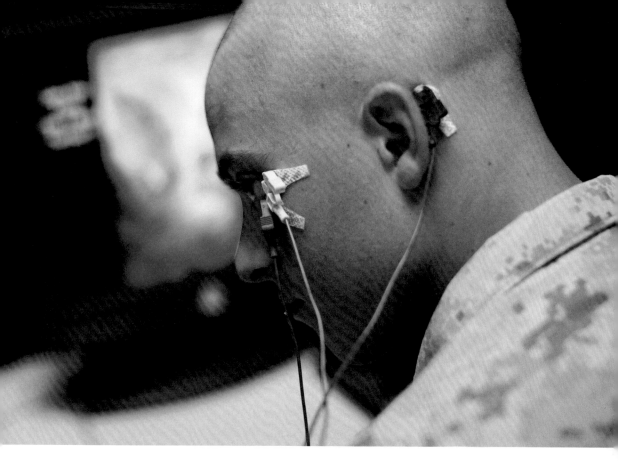

men who served in Vietnam had suffered PTSD at some point. This number astounded many, particularly since only 20% of veterans had been assigned to combat units.

Apparently, some type of amplification of symptoms was going on, to put it charitably. This issue was taken up in another article in this issue, bluntly entitled "Pseudo-PTSD," by [Drs. Gerald Rosen and Steven Taylor]. They note that PTSD is particularly vulnerable to malingering, both because the diagnosis is so often used in litigation, and because the symptom checklist is easily memorized and easily feigned. Clinicians are often fooled: in one study, even when clinicians were made aware of the possibility of malingering, many were unable to tell "real" from "fake" PTSD. Nobody knows how common malingered PTSD is, but the authors cite the forensic expert Philip Resnick's estimate that it is as high as 50% of all PTSD presentations.

Wearing sensors, this U.S. Marine undergoes a psychological test designed specifically to determine—before an individual ships out for active duty—whether he or she may be vulnerable to developing post-traumatic stress disorder. (AP Images)

The Future of PTSD

So where does this leave us? Are we to abandon the PTSD diagnosis altogether? Certainly not—[there are] patients who are clearly suffering some type of posttraumatic syndrome, and for these patients the category is needed, both for diagnosis and for directing treatment decisions. Furthermore, patients who have suffered trauma often find the PTSD criteria reassuring, since they help to normalize their reactions.

The final article offers some suggestions. Written by the folks who "invented" the original *DSM-3* PTSD diagnosis (including Robert Spitzer and Michael First), it suggests some significant tightening up of the diagnosis for the upcoming *DSM-V 21:233-241)*. The definition of trauma would require "*directly* experiencing" rather than simply "experiencing" an event; some of the more non-specific symptom criteria would be eliminated (including insomnia, irritability, poor concentration, and diminished interest); and the definitions of some core symptoms like flashbacks and avoidance would be changed to sound more extreme, in order to prevent people with milder symptoms from being included in the diagnosis.

In addition, a new "V" code would be introduced, entitled "Acute Stress Reaction," for patients who have suffered some sort of trauma, but whose symptoms are not at the severity required for PTSD.

A More Cautious Approach

None of these changes are certain, however. The *DSM-V* is just entering the workgroup phase and the new PTSD criteria won't be published until 2011. And some would argue that eliminating the "non-specific" criteria would actually detract from the validity of the diagnosis, since it is clear that so many patients suffer from them.

The bottom line is that in some people, trauma is associated with severe symptoms. The most useful aspect of these controversial articles is that they encourage us to be more thorough and cautious as we probe for PTSD symptoms And no one would argue with that.

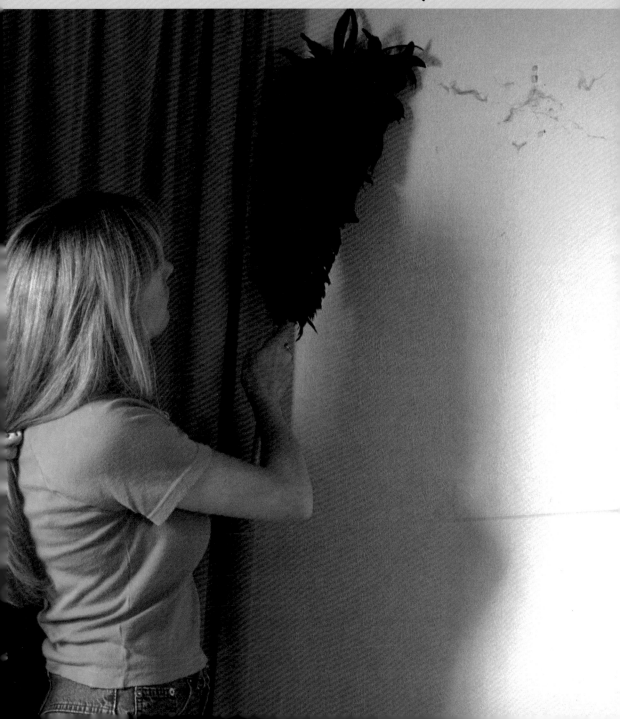

Living with Agoraphobia

Shirley B.

In this story Shirley B. shares her personal experience as an agoraphobic (one who fears being in public places). The goal for Shirley in sharing her story is that it may help others cope with the fear and shame of living with this disorder. Shirley explains how her agoraphobia happened gradually, but by the time she realized something was wrong she was too ashamed to tell anyone what she was feeling. As her seclusion deepened, Shirley would venture out of her home only for medical emergencies, and even then with enormous fear and trepidation. It was during one of these emergencies that her dentist recognized some of her physical symptoms and recommended that she seek professional help. Shirley then expresses her gratitude for all the people who helped her through the slow process of feeling as though she could face the world again. Shirley has omitted her last name from this story in order to maintain her privacy.

Photo on previous page. Some people who suffer from obsessive-compulsive disorder are consumed with a perpetual need to clean their homes. (© Angela Hampton Picture Library/Alamy)

SOURCE: Shirley B., "The Story of an Agoraphobic," Anxiety Disorders Association of America, ADAA.org, 2009. Copyright © 2009 Anxiety Disorders Association of America. Reproduced by permission.

As I am writing this I am a 46-year-old recovering agoraphobic. Whew! I never thought I could say that, let alone write it. But three weeks after I first admitted it in therapy, I crossed the street eight times on my own. Some people would say "That is no big deal." No, it's not a big deal—it's a MIRACLE! I wanted to shout, "Hello again world, I'm back. It's me, Shirley B!!!" Living is what I do now. Not as fully as I plan to, but it is so much more than just being. I am still struggling but that's okay. It took some time to be where I was, and it will take some time to get to where I am going. I look forward to the future. I have plans. I hope this article helps someone suffering from agoraphobia, or helps someone to understand what agoraphobia is.

There isn't much I can say about how I became agoraphobic. I just slipped a little day by day. When I noticed something was wrong, I didn't know how to stop it, and I was ashamed to ask for help for fear that someone would know my secret. I was ashamed to yell or scream for help, so I slipped and slipped away, deeper into my shell, my well, my pain. I wanted to talk, but I was ashamed to say some of the things that were on my mind. I did not want to be judged. I hid in my home and inside myself. I really wanted to find a big rock and hide under it. I neglected my health and ceased to care for myself. I hurt so deeply in my heart and soul that I felt the pain would never end. I thought life was something for other people, not for me. My understanding of existence was just to be, nothing more than just to be.

Fear of Going Out

My daughter Nadeen was always by my side on those rare occasions when I ventured outside, forced to leave my home when I needed medical attention. In the past my fear kept me at home with all sorts of physical pains and ailments, as horrific as the pain was, the pain of facing the outside world was greater. When I had two

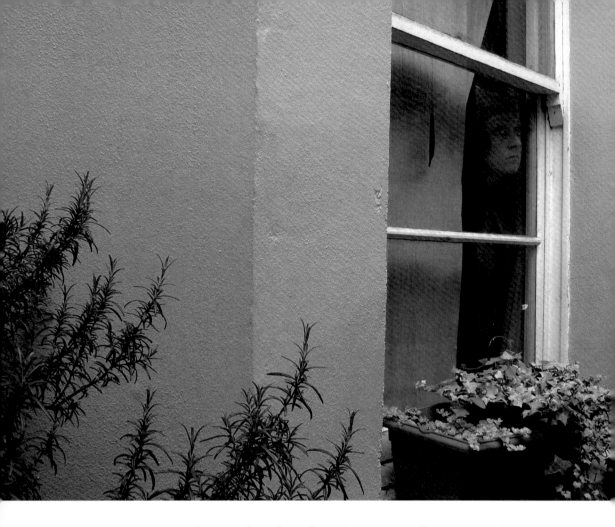

People with agoraphobia have a deeply rooted fear of venturing outside their homes. (**Karen Brett/ Photo Researchers, Inc.**)

abscessed teeth and my jaw was swollen to twice its normal size I was in such excruciating pain that I had to go to the dentist. So with my legs wobbling, my heart pounding, my hands sweating, and my throat choking, to the dentist I went. After examining my x-rays, the dentist said he wouldn't be able to do anything with my teeth because they were so infected, he prescribed medication for the pain and infection and said that I must return in ten days, not in two years. I felt as though those ten days were a countdown to my own execution. Each day passed at lightning speed—like a clock ticking away. The fear grew stronger and stronger. I had to walk around with my hand on my heart to keep it from jumping so hard, as if I were pledging allegiance, which

PERSPECTIVES ON DISEASES AND DISORDERS

I was—to my fears and phobia. I asked God to please give me strength to go back to the dentist. When the day came, I knew that my preparations would take me a little over four hours. I had to leave time, not just to bathe and dress, but to debate with myself about going.

When the dentist saw me, I was sweating profusely and trembling. He spoke with me for a few minutes, explaining what he was going to do, and said that I should relax. He also said that he felt I was depressed and maybe I should talk with someone about it. I don't know how he knew, but he knew. I was being found out. My secret was not as safe as I thought it was. I thought about how three months earlier my medical doctor had also said that I seemed depressed. He thought that perhaps I should be on some antidepressants. Unfortunately, antidepressants were not the answer for me. I felt hopeless again until Dr. L. told me that people can be treated in many different ways, there were several options and not to lose hope. There were other forms of treatment.

Getting Help

I thought that I didn't know where to begin, not realizing that wanting to change was a beginning itself, my first step toward recovery. I told my daughter that I needed help. She looked at me with love and tears in her eyes and said "Mom, I'm trying to help you in every way I know how. I don't know what else I can do." I told her that I needed a professional to show me how to help myself.

I was shaking so badly as I went to meet Dr. Beth Halpern that Nadeen had to hold my arm, but I also felt hopeful. Dr. Halpern and I talked for quite awhile. I couldn't believe that I was saying all the things that I was saying. I found myself asking her questions, such as: "Do you think I can be helped?" She said "yes." I decided to ask the question that frightened me most of all. I asked if she thought I was crazy. Dr. Halpern bent toward me and said, "Shirley, you are not crazy, you are not crazy." I smiled and sighed with relief.

As I write these words on paper, my heart fills with gratitude for all the people who have helped me towards my recovery. My first therapist, Jennifer Cantor, helped me lay the foundation for all of the therapy to follow. She had to actually teach me how to breathe properly, which is essential to relaxation. I know that after each session I had with Ms. Cantor, I walked away feeling stronger. At the end of our sessions Ms. Cantor gave me a homework assignment. My final assignment was to make a list of all the accomplishments I had made since starting treatment. I started my list and before I knew it I had written nearly to the end of the page: going to the supermarket alone, riding a bus, going to therapy and returning home alone. I felt proud and strong, but at the same time I realized that I still had work to do.

FAST FACT

The National Health Service of the United Kingdom estimates that between 4 and 5 percent of the population is affected by panic disorder and agoraphobia.

No More Hiding

I began my treatment with my new and current therapist, Ms. Alex Bloom. Ms. Bloom suggested that I come up with one thing that I would like to do. I had an idea of what that might be—writing an article about my treatment. Ms. Bloom thought is was a fantastic idea.

I wasn't scared on the subway that day (not very much anyway) as I thought about writing my article. I realized that I was smiling. Each week that followed I had at least two chapters written. I would start each session by reading the chapters I had written. Ms. Bloom said she could tell that my writing was helping me and she felt sure it would be of some help to others. She said that perhaps we could get my story typed and distributed to some people—it might help. I was overjoyed. Ms. Bloom's faith in me and in what I was doing was invaluable. If you are reading this, then my wish has become a reality. I hope this helps someone—anyone—in some way.

I no longer hide inside that deep dark hiding place, but my struggle continues. There are more challenges to conquer. I will not hide any longer in the shadow. I choose to walk toward my fears with the strength of the accomplishments I have made and with faith in my heart.

A College Student Struggles with Obsessive-Compulsive Disorder

Huw Davies

Huw Davies is a young writer working toward a postgraduate diploma in magazine journalism from Cardiff University in the United Kingdom. In this article Davies reveals his personal struggles with obsessive-compulsive disorder and explains some of his compulsive behaviors. For example, he washes his hands forty to fifty times a day. He has a tendency to count everything, including the words he speaks, often trying to create patterns of words that are divisible by three. Huw also has a habit of counting the words of people that are talking to him, which, he acknowledges, sometimes makes him appear rude. He worries about his compulsion with counting words, which also has made its way into his typing and writing, and wonders what effect it might have on his future as a journalist. However, Davies is waiting to begin cognitive-behavioral therapy, and is hopeful about the future.

People often talk about how hard it is to write. The words don't come, they say. Their mind goes blank. It's frustrating. People talk less often about how hard it is to literally write something. To type without backspacing needlessly, deleting and rewriting, deleting and rewriting, addingt letterss to thea end of wordsa, highlighting text for no reason, reading what you've written aloud until the words make no sense and having to include random lemon words because . . . well, you just have to. That's frustrating.

I suffer from Obsessive-Compulsive Disorder (OCD). My afflictions are mild and, to an extent, controllable. They're inconvenient, not incapacitating. I count everything, I wash my hands 40 to 50 times a day, I sometimes have to turn certain ways. When writing I suffer the obsessive compulsions mentioned above—though, obviously, equally obsessive editing prevents my written work reading like the last paragraph. These difficulties haven't taken over my life. I'm one of the lucky ones.

Among others, Jessica Alba, Paul Gascoigne and Cameron Diaz have all confessed to having some form of OCD. Diaz's case is particularly interesting: not dissimilarly to multimillionaire entrepreneur Howard Hughes, she opens doors with elbows to avoid touching supposedly germ-infested doorknobs. This may seem overly paranoid, but to Diaz and other contamination OCD sufferers, it is necessary.

Issues with Counting

[Soccer star] David Beckham, meanwhile, admits to an obsession with symmetry. In fact, his wife Victoria admitted it for him; in her own, inimitable words: "He's got that obsessive-compulsive thing." She explained how their fridges are coordinated, saying, "Everything is symmetrical. If there's three cans of Diet Coke, he'd throw one away rather than having three—because it has to be an even number."

This suggests that Beckham has issues with counting as well as symmetry. Counting is a common affliction for OCD sufferers, and perhaps my own biggest problem. Sufferers count to ensure there is the "right" number of something. For Beckham it's cans of drink in a fridge; for others, it's pens lined up on a table, coins in a pocket or even bricks in a wall (although obviously this one isn't changeable—merely "countable").

For (1) me, (2) it's (3) words (4). For some time now I've found myself unable to stop counting the number of words being said in a conversation, in my speech and in others'. Usually they have to be divisible by three. Sometimes five. Either way, it makes me add extra words when I'm talking, to make up the numbers. Sherbert. Fortunately, I talk too much to be able to count after a while.

Unfortunately, counting other people's words while they're talking can make me appear extremely rude. Not because I'm counting them out loud—that really would be rude—but because I find it difficult to concentrate on what they are saying, which can be very noticeable. Double the effect if there is a brick wall in the background, as I find myself counting its patterns. As someone who loves conversation, I hate not being able to immerse myself in it.

Typing Compulsions

Conversing with me was difficult when I was a child, too, but for a very different reason: I never stopped talking. I don't think I had OCD then. I certainly never noticed it. A counsellor told me she believed it nearly always stemmed from a traumatic childhood experience. This is a popular theory, perhaps because it's the most exciting one. But no, I didn't fall into a bog when I was seven or anything like that. I just noticed it at university, and then that it was steadily worsening. On average, the condition affects women in their early 20s and men in late adolescence.

As anyone who saw [the British television soap opera] *Hollyoaks*' brief flirtation with an OCD storyline will know, it can affect students massively. Living in student housing doesn't help anyone with cleanliness issues, let alone contamination OCD. My own particular brand of the condition decided to target my university work; essays became even more of a chore than usual.

As well as the aforementioned typing compulsions, I couldn't move on to another paragraph without knowing the one before it was word-perfect. In fact, comma-perfect: I would spend several hours debating in my head, and to anyone who would listen, whether part of a sentence required a hyphen or a semi-colon.

I'm not detailing my condition to be labelled "weird" by anyone reading, or for personal attention. On the contrary, it's very difficult to admit to having it. Even if my typing compulsions have improved—or, more accurately, my OCD has moved more prominently into other areas such as cleanliness and counting—how do I tell future employers about the problems I've had with working efficiently? Will telling people about my condition hold me back? I want to be a journalist—but could this, written at the age of 21, be the last article I ever have printed?

> **FAST FACT**
>
> According to the Web site Understanding Obsessive-Compulsive Disorder, surveys estimate that less than 10 percent of those suffering with OCD are currently in treatment.

Drawing Attention to the Disorder

It is hard to shake these anxieties. I am probably lucky that mine revolve around only my career. For others, the prospect of one's relationship with others changing upon "coming out" with OCD can be terrifying.

It is easy to feel as if you are the only person who suffers from such strange thoughts and urges. I also didn't know how debilitating it can be (some sufferers are confined to their bedrooms and wash their hands several hundred times every day). I am thankful that my condition is not more severe. In fact, I often feel guilty explaining it to people, knowing there are others with much worse experiences. But this is not the right way to look at an illness; after all, saying you feel down isn't

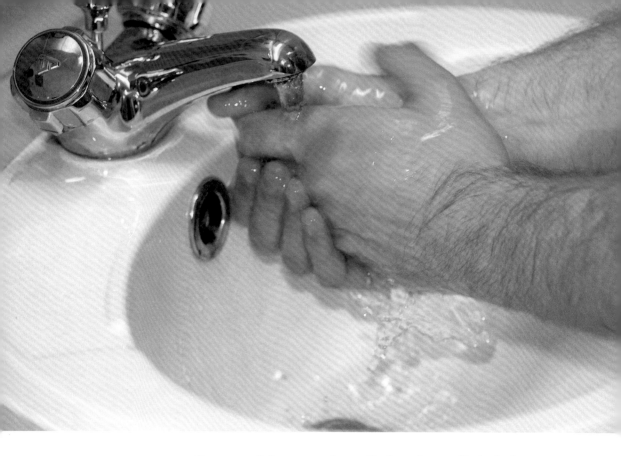

Some who suffer with obsessive-compulsive disorder are compelled to wash their hands over two hundred times a day. (Crown Copyright courtesy of Central Science Laboratory/Photo Researchers, Inc.)

disrespectful to people suffering from clinical depression. Sometimes you just have to consider your own problems.

I am not looking for sympathy. I am simply trying to draw attention to some of the many different forms of OCD. When it comes to this disorder, there are obsessions and there are compulsions. The stereotypes— handwashing, checking and so on—are compulsions: thoughts, or more commonly actions, that a person sees as necessary to reduce anxiety. These can be based on (sometimes skewed) logic or superstition, and are often recognised by the sufferer to be irrational. Carrying them out, however, alleviates concern, even when they are completely unrelated to an anxiety—for example, turning around three times will not prevent the roof falling in, but the fact that it does not "confirms" the compulsion's efficacy. It is not unlike taking a placebo.

Finding Help

Obsessions—recurrent thoughts, ideas or images—can take on very disturbing forms; forms the sufferer would consciously never think of entertaining, such as killing a relative. Regular superstitious rituals can arise from the desire to make up for such thoughts.

Often these are based on apparent logic albeit exaggerated—for example, Diaz's attempt to avoid germs on doorknobs—but many are irrational. These include everyday superstitions: for example, seeing a solitary magpie may trigger an obsession over a loved one dying ("One for sorrow, two for joy", etc); saluting the magpie to prevent this is an immediate compulsion. I'm not alone in touching wood, but I don't see it as a superstition, it's an automatic compulsion.

Obviously this doesn't mean everyone with a superstition has OCD; simply that it is more understandable than some may think. Sadly, this leads many to underestimate the potentially devastating power of the condition.

I have only recently come out about my own OCD, and my doctor, who was very understanding, put me on a waiting list for cognitive behavioural therapy (CBT). But although this is thought to be the best way to tackle OCD, discussing experiences is a good way to start, and OCD Action runs support groups for sufferers. I have also been trying one element of CBT myself—exposure and response prevention—which entails exposing oneself to an anxiety-inducing discomfort and resisting the usual "escape response." For example, a sufferer with cleanliness issues could plant his hands in some mud, and attempt to resist the urge to clean them. As yet, I have not been overly successful because I still have the mindset that "It's OK, because soon I will be washing myself clean." I hope to have improved by the time I commence my CBT with a professional at hand.

Support of Friends and Family

Luckily, my family and friends have been supportive of my OCD, although sadly many blame it on themselves, although it is simply not their fault. Still, it is heartening that they care; it is important for non-sufferers to be understanding, even if they don't understand. To anyone who takes offence at seeing the rim of a glass wiped after they've used it, it really is nothing personal; it may seem hard to believe, but it's not. And to anyone who actually licks the rim of the glass out of protest—well, that's just not very nice, is it?

Perhaps the most important thing is for sufferers not to feel ashamed. One great obstacle to seeking therapy is thinking, "But this is who I am." I know I've felt that. But it's not. It's Obsessive-Compulsive Disorder. When you have the notion in your head of taking a knife to your nearest and dearest, that is OCD; but while you continue to reject that notion, that is you, and you're a lot healthier than you think.

And you know what? As long as it's under control, a little bit of eccentricity is not such a bad thing (21).

Fighting Panic Disorder Is a Lifelong Battle

Harriet Brown

In this article Harriet Brown relates her lifelong struggle with panic disorder. She describes what it feels like when she has a panic attack—a pounding heart, the feeling of being suffocated. She writes that the current thinking concerning panic disorder is that it has a biological connection, which means that genetics plays a major role in who gets the disorder. She has gone through some talk therapy, and though it helped her in other ways, it did not curb her panic attacks. She went on antidepressants, and they helped but had detrimental side effects. She went off the medication and tried cognitive-behavioral therapy, but that also proved ineffective. Brown still struggles with attacks but hopes that if a biological source can be proven, it may change the way society looks at those with panic disorder. Brown is an author living in Syracuse, New York, where she teaches magazine journalism at Syracuse University.

I'm driving to work on a picture-perfect summer day—blue sky, puffy clouds, Warren Zevon on the CD player—when it starts. Somewhere toward the end of "Lawyers, Guns, and Money," my heart begins to flutter, just a little, a skipped beat here and there. Soon, instead of its usual steady lub-dub, it's knocking in chaotic, syncopated bursts. The air in the car thickens, gets stuffy; I inhale deeply, trying to pull in more air, but I can't get enough. I'm suffocating, right here in my own car. Now my heart's pounding hard and fast, and my hands on the steering wheel are slick with sweat. A feeling of terror blooms in my chest, exploding into every cell of my body.

I pull over, hit the power-lock button, and close my eyes. My hands shake, and my breath comes in short, panicked gasps. Everything in me wants to open the door and run away from the car, away from this small and terrible space. Away from the sick, disoriented feeling that's racing through my body.

I feel like I'm about to die. But I know, somewhere inside the adrenaline fog, that I'm not dying. I know that this is a panic attack, one of thousands I've had in my life. If I sit here long enough—five minutes, ten, 20—my heart will eventually slow down, my breath come more evenly. And I've also been through this enough to know that this is just the beginning, the first salvo of many. The thought triggers another run of palpitations as I know that I'm in for days, weeks, maybe months of attacks like this.

A Lifetime of Attacks

Most people have one, maybe two panic attacks in their lives. But for an unlucky few, the first attack leads to a lifetime of them. Mine started when I was about eight years old. I was afraid of everything—matches, being locked in the bathroom, burglars, choking, dogs, airplanes. Fear spilled into every corner of my life. During the day, I could usually distract myself with school, piano, books. But once the lights went out, I was alone and vulnerable. I lay awake each night for hours, waves of fear washing through my body. At times I felt unreal, as if I were standing outside myself and looking back at a stranger.

The fear set me apart from others, making me into something of a loner. I knew I couldn't tell other kids how I was feeling; they would think I was crazy. I thought I was crazy, that the fear and the feelings were all my fault, and so I hid them from other people. I tried to tell my parents once. "You think too much," my mother responded. "Try not to worry," advised my father, himself a consummate worrier.

I was an adult before I had a name for what was wrong with me: panic disorder. The word *panic* comes from Pan, the Greek god who was thought to make mysterious sounds that caused "unreasoning fear." The fear that marks a panic attack is both quantitatively and qualitatively different from fears that are rooted in reality. It comes on suddenly, a lightning strike of physiological and psychological symptoms: rapid heartbeat, sweating, chest pain, shortness of breath, hyperventilation, dizziness, feelings of unreality, terror, and obsessive thinking. I've had them all—and sometimes all at once.

Running in the Family

Nearly 5 percent of the U.S. population meets the diagnostic criteria for panic disorder, having at least one panic attack a month. Many go on to develop agoraphobia, a fear of panic attacks themselves that makes them constrict their activities, often to the point of being unable to leave their homes. Women are twice as likely as men to develop the illness, which probably explains why sufferers have historically been considered nervous, excitable, or insane. I'd guess that many "nervous breakdowns" are actually bouts of panic disorder.

The current thinking on panic disorder, as on depression, eating disorders, and other mental illnesses, is that it is biological. "There's something we inherit that makes some people more vulnerable to panic attacks and anxiety about having more attacks," says David Barlow, Ph.D., director of the Center for Anxiety and Related Disorders at Boston University. "If you have the genes, you might be more likely to have a panic attack. You might get more anxious about it if you do have one. It lowers the threshold." Panic disorder runs in families; if you've got a parent or sibling with it, you're up to eight times more likely to develop it yourself. (One of my daughters also has panic disorder.)

For some people, the attacks remain discrete, self-limiting episodes of fear. For others, like me, one attack can morph into a prolonged reign of terror. Everyone has her own triggers—stress, hormonal shifts, and specific phobias like heights and tight spaces are among the most common. For me, these can be as simple as drinking too much coffee and having palpitations, or as complex as anticipating a fearful situation—a confrontation at work, a medical procedure. Either way, there's nothing subtle about a panic attack. It comes on like a freight train, immersing me in an unpleasantly altered state of reality. Adrenaline flows, heart rate increases, and the body gets ready to either fight the threat or run away. In the case of panic disorder, though, the fight-or-flight instinct is a liability not a survival mechanism, because the danger is internal rather than external. You can't run from the fear when it's inside your own body and mind. You can't fight or think your way out of it. You can only endure.

State of Terror

One of my worst bouts with panic disorder began when I moved to New York City after college. On the first day of my first job—the beginning of my life as an adult—I rode the elevator to the thirty-third floor and met my new boss at the reception desk. As she led me toward her office, I felt the room suddenly pitch, as if I were on a boat in the middle of a violent sea. A rush of physical dizziness swept over me as my heart started to pound. My boss was still talking, and I was trying to be bright and enthusiastic, but inside I was freaking out. I wanted to fall down on the floor and cry. I wanted to run.

God knows what my boss thought of me, then or in the months that followed, as the panic attacks came ten and 20 a day and I tried to function in a constant state of terror. I'd wake every morning and feel fine for a minute or two. Then the switch would get flipped; the fear would kick in, and nothing I thought or felt or did could stop it.

Those episodes propelled me to seek out the first of many therapists. Once a week for an hour I'd talk about my panic attacks, my childhood, my family. I learned a lot about myself. But talk therapy didn't make the attacks stop. Over the next decade, my panic disorder waxed and waned. When I got pregnant at age 31, it suddenly, blessedly, went away—which is not unusual, according to David Barlow. It stayed dormant for nearly five years, through breast-feeding, a miscarriage, and another pregnancy.

I thought I was cured. But the day after my second daughter was born, the panic began all over again. After a month I finally got in to see a psychiatrist, who prescribed an SSRI [selective serotonin reuptake inhibitor]. Within three weeks of starting it, I felt normal once more.

This makes sense, explains Alexander Neumeister, M.D., an associate professor of psychiatry at Yale University School of Medicine, because drugs like Zoloft affect both of the major neurotransmitters that play a role in panic disorder. SSRIs raise available levels of serotonin in the brain, which in turn affects levels of norepinephrine.

> **FAST FACT**
>
> Panic disorder typically strikes in young adulthood. Roughly half of all people who have panic disorder develop the condition before age twenty-four.

"If you don't have enough serotonin, this system gets out of control and starts to function without regulation," says Neumeister. The result is the kind of roller coaster of physiological and psychological symptoms I've experienced.

While the antidepressant kept my panic disorder at bay, it had two unfortunate side effects: I gained weight, and I was unable to write. After five years I stopped taking the drugs. The writing came back, and so did the panic disorder.

Cognitive Behavioral Therapy

I was older by then, better at coping with the attacks but more determined not to spend so much of my life in misery. I knew I had to do something different. One option was a trip to the Center for Anxiety and Related Disorders in Boston for a course of Cognitive Behavioral Therapy. The three-part treatment teaches people to understand, tolerate, and eventually master their fears. "They learn at an emotional level what they know at a rational level, that they're harmless sensations," explains Barlow, who now directs the center. Up to 80 percent of those who go through the treatment program have "a very good response," according to Barlow, who's currently working on a project to help teens with panic disorder.

There's no question that the disorder tends to be chronic, something people must learn to manage rather than cure. At the moment, Cognitive Behavioral Therapy is the treatment of choice, in part because a 2003 paper published in the journal *Depression and Anxiety* showed that it has a "modest protective effect" against relapse.

I've done a little CBT over the years, but I didn't find it effective, maybe because my panic attacks are usually triggered by hormonal shifts, coming on as I entered puberty, going away with pregnancy, returning with perimenopause. I now carry lorazepam, an antianxiety medicine, and use it at the first sign of an attack. With the help of a good psychiatrist, I've learned that if I can stop the cycle of adrenaline and anxiety early, it doesn't build into the kind of months-long nightmare I experienced in my teens and 20s.

The Biological Basis

Sometimes I still miss the early-warning signs, confusing the beginning of an attack with an asthma attack or worse. "People with panic disorder often end up in the emergency room for heart tests," says Rob Philibert, M.D., Ph.D., associate professor of psychiatry at the University of Iowa Roy J. and Lucille A. Carver College of Medicine. I've been there and done that, feeling ashamed but relieved to be told I'm "only" having panic attack.

Philibert says he's close to developing a blood test to screen for panic disorder. Such a test would underscore the biological basis of the disorder and would mark a profound change in the way the medical profession sees people with panic disorder—and how we see ourselves.

My life has been shaped by fear, by the coping strategies I developed to deal with it—some good, some unhealthy—and by my sense of being alone and crazy. How would I be different if, say, my parents had been able to take me to a doctor for a blood test and a diagnosis? I can't help wondering how much of my life has literally been consumed by the obsessive thoughts and fears that succeeded one another like waves on a beach: I was having a heart attack; I had a brain tumor; I was losing my mind.

For a long time I felt bitter about all that I've lost to panic disorder. But I've come to understand that I've gained some, too. I've had to work to attain something other people take for granted: a sense of equilibrium, which comes in part from understanding that I'm not alone. And that my life is about a lot more than fear.

GLOSSARY

agoraphobia An abnormal and persistent fear of public places or open areas, especially those from which escape could be difficult or help not immediately accessible.

antidepressant A term typically used to describe medications that are used in the treatment of depression. Such medications are sometimes found useful in the treatment of anxiety disorder.

anxiety A sense of apprehension and fear often marked by physical symptoms such as sweating, tension, and increased heart rate.

anxiety disorder A chronic condition characterized by an excessive and persistent sense of apprehension with physical symptoms such as sweating, palpitations, and feelings of stress. Anxiety disorders have biological and environmental causes.

anxiolytics The medications that reduce the symptoms of anxiety.

behavior therapy The treatment used to help patients substitute desirable responses and behavior patterns for undesirable ones.

benzodiazepines A class of drugs that act as tranquilizers and are commonly used in the treatment of anxiety.

beta blockers A class of drugs typically used to decrease blood pressure and also prescribed to ease physical symptoms of anxiety associated with social phobia.

cognitive-behavioral therapy A relatively short-term form of psychotherapy based on the concept that the way we think about things affects how we feel emotionally. Cognitive therapy focuses on present thinking, behavior, and communication rather than on past experiences and is oriented toward problem solving.

comorbidity The coexistence of two or more disease processes.

compulsion	An irrational motive for performing trivial or repetitive actions, even against one's will.
depression	A biologically based psychological disorder marked by sadness, inactivity, difficulty with thinking and concentration, significant increase or decrease in appetite and sleep, feelings of dejection and hopelessness, and sometimes suicidal thoughts or actions.
direct conditioning	Exposure to an early traumatic event that may have an impact on the development of social anxiety, sometimes years later.
DSM-IV	The fourth edition of *Diagnostic and Statistical Manual of Mental Disorders (DSM)*, a comprehensive classification of officially recognized psychiatric disorders. *DSM-IV* was issued in 1993.
exposure therapy	A type of treatment that includes gradually bringing patients into contact with a feared object or situation. Patients learn that the object or situation can be faced and that avoidance is unnecessary.
family therapy	The efforts aimed at helping a patient's family understand and cope with the patient's disorder and help in the patient's recovery.
generalized anxiety disorder	A condition characterized by six months or more of chronic, exaggerated worry and tension that is unfounded or much more severe than the normal anxiety most people experience. Physical symptoms, such as headache, fatigue, nausea, and insomnia, are often exhibited by sufferers.
genetically predisposed	The potential for an individual to develop a condition or trait because of its presence in a family member.
hoarding	The compulsive acquisition of and failure to use or discard such a large number of seemingly useless possessions that it causes significant clutter and impairment to basic living activities such as mobility, cooking, cleaning, showering, or sleeping.
neurosis	A long-term disorder featuring anxiety and/or exaggerated behavior dedicated to avoiding anxiety. Sufferers understand that the condition is abnormal.

neurotransmitter	A chemical substance released by nerve cell endings to transmit impulses across the space between nerve cells, tissues, or organs.
obsessive-compulsive disorder	A condition marked by persistent and recurring thoughts (obsessions) typically reflecting exaggerated anxiety or fears that have no basis in reality. Sufferers often feel compelled to perform a ritual or routine to help relieve anxiety caused by their obsessions.
panic disorder	A condition characterized by feelings of extreme fear and dread that strike unexpectedly and repeatedly for no apparent reason, often accompanied by intense physical symptoms, such as chest pain, pounding heart, shortness of breath, dizziness, or abdominal distress.
pharmacotherapy	The treatment of a disease or disorder with drugs.
phobia	An intense and persistent fear of certain situations, activities, things, or people. The main symptom of this disorder is the excessive and unreasonable desire to avoid the feared subject.
post-traumatic stress disorder	A condition that results from experiencing or witnessing an unusually distressing event. Symptoms range from repeatedly reliving the trauma, such as in dreams or flashbacks, to general emotional numbness, which often causes sufferers to withdraw from family and friends.
psychotherapy	An intentional, interpersonal relationship used by trained psychotherapists to aid a client or patient in problems of living. Psychotherapists employ a range of techniques based on experiential relationship building, dialogue, communication, and behavior change.
selective serotonin reuptake inhibitors (SSRIs)	A class of antidepressants used in the treatment of depression, anxiety disorders, and some personality disorders.
separation anxiety disorder	The feeling of excessive and inappropriate levels of anxiety over being separated from a person or place. Separation anxiety itself is a normal part of development in babies or children, and it is only when this feeling is excessive or inappropriate that it can be considered a disorder.

side effect	A secondary and usually adverse effect of a drug or therapy.
social anxiety disorder	A condition characterized by intense anxiety of being judged by others and/or publicly behaving in a way that could lead to embarrassment or ridicule.
tricyclic antidepressants (TCAs)	A class of antidepressants useful in treating some anxiety disorders.

CHRONOLOGY

1844   Søren Kierkegaard publishes *The Concept of Anxiety*, which is commonly thought of as the first wide-ranging explanation of anxiety.

1923   Mary Cover Jones conducts a study on Peter, a child with a fear of white rabbits. She uses "direct conditioning" to gradually alleviate his fears.

1949   Australian psychiatrist J.F.J. Cade introduces the use of lithium to treat psychosis. Before this, drugs had been used mostly to sedate patients but were ineffective in treating their symptoms.

1952   The American Psychiatric Association (APA) publishes the first *Diagnostic and Statistical Manual of Mental Disorders (DSM)*, creating the modern classification system for mental disorders.

mid-1950s   Behavior therapy is developed, which holds that patients with phobias can overcome their fears through training and conditioning.

1959   Developed by M. Hamilton, the Hamilton Anxiety Scale (Ham-A) measures the severity of a patient's anxiety.

1960s   Aaron T. Beck develops a system of psychotherapy called "Cognitive Therapy."

1976   Beck publishes *Cognitive Therapy and the Emotional Disorders.* In this book Beck expands his focus to include anxiety disorders.

1980   A group of clinicians and patients form the Phobia Society of America (PSA).

The American Psychiatric Association publishes its *Diagnostic and Statistical Manual of Mental Disorders-III* (*DSM-III*), which differentiates anxiety disorders into specific illnesses.

1984   *Newsweek* publishes a landmark cover story on phobias. The article cites studies that show a link between abnormal blood flow in the brain and panic attacks.

1986   A National Institute of Mental Health (NIMH) study shows that panic disorder is linked to serious social and health consequences similar to or greater than those associated with significant depression.

1987   The Phobia Society of America testifies before the U.S. House of Representatives to describe the nature, seriousness, and prevalence of anxiety disorders.

1990   The U.S. Food and Drug Administration (FDA) approves alprazolam (Xanax) to treat panic disorder.

Beck publishes the *Beck Anxiety Inventory (BAI) Manual,* which introduces a scale to test an individual's anxiety levels.

The Phobia Society of America becomes the Anxiety Disorders Association of America (ADAA).

1990–1992   The National Comorbidity Survey (NCS) of the United States is conducted. It was the first large-scale field study of mental health in the nation. The NCS was designed to assess mental disorders based on the updated disease categories in the revised *Diagnostic and Statistical Manual of Mental Disorders-III-R* (*DSM-III-R*).

1991   A panel of experts is convened by the NIMH to determine the epidemiology, natural history, and course of panic disorder. They are also tasked with evaluating the effectiveness of cognitive-behavioral therapy and medications.

1994   The FDA approves the first selective serotonin reuptake inhibitor (SSRI), fluoxetine (Prozac), to treat obsessive-compulsive disorder (OCD).

1997   The Anxiety Disorders Association of America funds a study that finds that the annual cost of anxiety disorders in the United States is more than 42 billion dollars.

2005   Researchers study a new nationally representative sample of the U.S. population, repeating many of the questions from the original National Comorbidity Survey and expanding the study's scope by incorporating updated disease assessment criteria based on the *Diagnostic and Statistical Manual of Mental Disorders-IV* (*DSM-III*).

ORGANIZATIONS TO CONTACT

The editors have compiled the following list of organizations concerned with the issues debated in this book. The descriptions are derived from materials provided by the organizations. All have publications or information available for interested readers. The list was compiled on the date of publication of the present volume; the information provided here may change. Be aware that many organizations take several weeks or longer to respond to inquiries, so allow as much time as possible.

American Psychiatric Association's Healthy Minds
1000 Wilson Blvd.
Ste. 1825, Arlington
VA 22209
(888) 357-7924
www.healthyminds.org

HealthyMinds.org is the American Psychiatric Association's online resource for anyone seeking mental health information. The American Psychiatric Association (APA) is a national medical specialty society whose physician members specialize in diagnosis, treatment, prevention, and research of mental illnesses. The APA publishes a series of brochures that are designed to improve mental health by promoting informed factual discussion of psychiatric disorders and their treatments.

American Psychological Association (APA)
750 First St. NE
Washington, DC
20002-4242
(800) 374-2721 or
(202) 336-5500
www.apa.org

The APA is a scientific and professional organization that represents psychology in the United States. The mission of the APA is to advance the creation, communication, and application of psychological knowledge to benefit society and improve people's lives. The APA publishes books, magazines, and online newsletters, all of which can be found through its Web site.

Anxiety Disorders Association of America (ADAA)
8730 Georgia Ave.
Ste., 600, Silver Spring
MD 20910
(240) 485-1001
fax: (240) 485-1035
www.adaa.org

The ADAA is a national nonprofit organization dedicated to the prevention, treatment, and cure of anxiety disorders and to improving the lives of all people who suffer from them. The association disseminates information, links people who need treatment with those who can provide it, and advocates for cost-effective treatments. The ADAA publishes books, downloadable brochures, and *Triumph,* an e-newsletter.

Association for Behavior Analysis International (ABAI)
550 W. Centre Ave.
Ste. 1, Portage, MI
49024-5364
(269) 492-9310
fax: (269) 492-9316
www.abainternational
.org

The ABAI is a nonprofit professional membership organization with the mission to contribute to the well-being of society by developing, enhancing, and supporting the growth and vitality of the science of behavior analysis through research, education, and practice. ABAI publishes a monthly newsletter and three scholarly journals.

Association for Behavioral and Cognitive Therapies (ABCT)
305 Seventh Ave.
16th Fl., New York
NY 10001
(212) 647-1890
fax: (212) 647-1865
www.abct.org

The ABCT is an interdisciplinary organization committed to the advancement of a scientific approach to the understanding of problems of the human condition. These aims are achieved through the investigation and application of behavioral, cognitive, and other evidence-based principles. ABCT offers an archive of fact sheets on its Web site that covers a wide array of mental health issues.

International OCD Foundation (IOCDF)
112 Water St., Ste. 501, Boston, MA 02109
(617) 973-5801
fax: (617) 973-5803
www.ocfoundation
.org

The IOCDF is an international nonprofit organization made up of people with obsessive-compulsive disorder (OCD) and related disorders, as well as their families, friends, professionals, and others. The foundation's mission is to educate the public about OCD, support research into the causes and treatment of OCD, improve access to resources, and advocate for the OCD community. IOCDF publishes books, downloadable brochures, and fact sheets that are available on its Web site.

Mental Health America
2000 N. Beauregard St., 6th Fl. Alexandria, VA 22311
(703) 684-7722, (800) 969-6642
fax: (703) 684-5968
www.mentalhealth
america.net

Mental Health America is dedicated to helping all people live mentally healthier lives. It represents a growing movement of Americans who promote mental wellness for the health and well-being of the nation—every day and in times of crisis. Mental Health America publishes books, brochures, videos, and a newsletter, the *Bell*.

National Alliance on Mental Illness (NAMI)
3803 N. Fairfax Dr. Ste. 100, Arlington VA 22203
(703) 524-7600
fax: (703) 524-9094
www.nami.org

NAMI is dedicated to improving the lives of individuals and families affected by mental illness. The alliance is a grassroots mental health advocacy organization that seeks to improve the lives of those with serious mental illnesses through research, education, and community support. NAMI publishes the *Advocate* magazine.

National Center for PTSD
810 Vermont Ave.
NW, Washington, DC
20420
(802) 296-6300
www.ptsd.va.gov

The National Center for PTSD is the center of excellence for research and education on the prevention, understanding, and treatment of post-traumatic stress disorder. Its purpose is to improve the well-being and understanding of American veterans. It conducts cutting edge research and applies resultant findings to advance the science and to promote the understanding of traumatic stress. The center's Web site includes fact sheets and videos about PTSD.

National Institute of Mental Health (NIMH)
6001 Executive Blvd.
Rm. 8184, MSC 9663
Bethesda, MD 20892-9663
(866) 615-9464
fax: (301) 443-4279
www.nimh.nih.gov

The National Institute of Mental Health is the U.S. government organization dedicated to transforming the understanding and treatment of mental illnesses through basic and clinical research, paving the way for prevention, recovery, and cure. NIMH publishes booklets, fact sheets, and easy-to-read topical introductions to mental health issues.

Screening for Mental Health Inc. (SMH)
One Washington St.
Ste. 304
Wellesley Hills, MA
02481
(781) 239-0071
fax: (781) 431-7447
ww.mentalhealth
screening.org

SMH is a nonprofit organization that develops and administers large-scale mental health screenings, including screenings for generalized anxiety disorder and post-traumatic stress disorder. Teaching people how to identify mental illness and specific ways to access treatment for themselves or a loved one is the cornerstone of SMH's programs. SMH publishes an online newsletter and offers the full archive on its Web site.

Sidran Institute
200 E. Joppa Rd.
Ste. 207, Baltimore
MD 21286-3107
(410) 825-8888
fax: (410) 337-0747
Web site: www.sidran
.org

Sidran Traumatic Stress Institute, Inc. is a nonprofit organization of international scope that helps people understand, recover from, and treat: traumatic stress (including PTSD), dissociative disorders, and co-occurring issues, such as addictions, self-injury, and suicidality. The institute publishes books and videos and offers several free, downloadable booklets online.

Social Phobia/Social Anxiety Association (SP/SAA)
2058 E. Topeka Dr.
Phoenix, AZ 85024
www.socialphobia.org

The SP/SAA, a nonprofit organization, was officially organized in 1997 to meet the growing needs of people throughout the world who have social phobia/social anxiety. The association provides support and information to those who suffer from social phobia, and hopes to educate friends and family members by offering practical examples of what life is like for people with social phobia. The organization publishes articles and fact sheets on its Web site.

Society for Neuroscience (SFN)
1121 Fourteenth St.
NW, Ste. 1010
Washington, DC
20005
(202) 962-4000
fax: (202) 962-4941
www.sfn.org

The SFN is a nonprofit membership organization of scientists and physicians who study the brain and nervous system. The society's mission is to advance the understanding of the brain and the nervous system, to provide professional developmental activities, and to promote the public's awareness of neuroscience. The SFN offers a number of publications in print and online, including *Brain Briefings*, a monthly newsletter.

FOR FURTHER READING

Books

Aaron T. Beck, Gary Emery, and Ruth Greenberg, *Anxiety Disorders and Phobias: A Cognitive Perspective.* New York: Basic Books, 2005.

Edmund J. Bourne, *The Anxiety & Phobia Workbook. 4th ed.* Oakland, CA: New Harbinger, 2005.

J. Paul Caldwell, *Anxiety Disorders: Everything You Need to Know.* Buffalo, NY: Firefly, 2005.

Carolyn Chambers Clark, *Living Well with Anxiety: What Your Doctor Doesn't Tell You . . . That You Need to Know.* New York: HarperPaperback, 2006.

Emily Ford, Michael Liebowitz, and Linda Wasmer Andrews, *What You Must Think of Me: A Firsthand Account of One Teenager's Experience with Social Anxiety Disorder.* New York: Oxford University Press, 2007.

John P. Forsyth and Georg H. Eifert, *The Mindfulness and Acceptance Workbook for Anxiety: A Guide to Breaking Free from Anxiety, Phobias, and Worry Using Acceptance and Commitment Therapy.* Oakland, CA: New Harbinger, 2008.

Stefan G. Hoffman and Michael W. Otto, *Cognitive Behavioral Therapy for Social Anxiety Disorder.* New York: Routledge, 2008.

Margaret Wehrenberg, *The Ten Best-Ever Anxiety Management Techniques: Understanding How Your Brain Makes You Anxious and What You Can Do to Change It.* New York: W.W. Norton, 2008.

Periodicals

Colby Buzzell, "Welcome Back: Three Years Out of the Army, Diagnosed with PTSD, I Recently Got a Nice Letter from the Pentagon Saying They'd Like Me Back in Iraq, Pronto. They Didn't Even Mind That I Was a Little Sick. And I'm Not the Only One," *Esquire,* September 2008.

Economist, "Stressed Out and Traumatized," March 5, 2005.

Lauren Russell Griffen, "When Panic Attacks," *Women's Health*, March 2008.

Steven E. Hyman, "Neuroscience: Obsessed with Grooming," *Nature*, August 23, 2007.

Ben Kallen, "Peace of Mind: If You Always Feel Anxious and Stressed, You May Have Generalized Anxiety Disorder. Here's How to Reclaim a Sense of Calm," *Natural Health*, December 2007.

Jeremy Katz, "Are You Crazy Enough to Succeed?" *Men's Health*, July/August 2008.

Jeffrey Kluger, "When Worry Hijacks the Brain," *Time*, August 13, 2007.

Meryl Davids Landau, "High Anxiety," *Ladies' Home Journal*, October 2009.

Mike Lipton, "Recipe for Living: Suffering from Acute Agoraphobia, TV Chef Paula Deen Cooked Up Her Own Cure," *People Weekly*, August 22, 2005.

Emily Listfield, "Fumbling Toward . . . Looking Out for . . . Diving into . . . Dreading . . . Feeling My Way to 40: What Mature 40-Something Is Afraid to Drive? Um, That Would Be Me," *Redbook*, May 2009.

Tim McGirk, "The Hell of PTSD," *Time*, November 30, 2009.

Elizabeth Roberts, "Are You Worrying Yourself Sick?" *Shape*, January 2009.

Roxanne Patel Shepelavy, "Extreme Stress: What Every Woman Should Know About Panic Attacks," *Good Housekeeping*, April 2009.

Abby Sher, "Diary of a Breakdown," *Self*, May 2007.

Matthew Shulman, "Being More than Merely Shy; Social Phobia Can Interfere with Work, Life, and Relationships," *U.S. News & World Report*, April 28, 2008.

INDEX